The Thre
The Brain

Are Psychiatrists
Necessary?

by

CHRISTOPHER HOSKIN

The June Press

The Author

Christopher Hoskin is the son of a distinguished cardiologist and has a degree in philosophy from Cambridge. In his early twenties he had mental troubles causing him to go to a psychoanalyst for many years. It was this growing awareness of the fate of others with mental problems that incited him to write this book.

June Press publications are not intended to represent a corporate view of developments in Psychology. They are to promote and develop ideas and encourage individuals to express views on all subjects, within the security and obligations of a stable and law-abiding nation. The views expressed in our publications are the sole responsibility of the authors.

First published in 2012

by The June Press Ltd

UK distributor
The June Press Ltd
PO Box 119
Totnes
Devon TQ9 7WA
Tel: 44(0)8456 120 175
Email: info@junepress.com
Web: www.junepress.com

ISBN 978-0-9534697-8-9

Contents

Acknowledgements

I wish to express my deepest gratitude to the many people who helped in the making of this book. My special thanks go to George Frankl, Naomi Davidov and Sheila Camino.

Christopher Hoskin, 2012

Introduction

This book is concerned with the treatment of mental illnesses by official psychiatry. It is not concerned with their treatment by psychotherapy, with which I have no quarrel, and which I approve of. Many, though by no means all, psychiatrists insist on treating mental illnesses as if they were no different from the illnesses and conditions treated in other branches of medicine. This has resulted in a vast amount of inappropriate treatment, often resulting in brain damage.

Of course, wrong or debilitating treatments do from time to time occur in ordinary medicine, where what is treated is some definite physical ailment. We can never exclude the possibility of bad treatment. But, in the case of psychiatry, there arise fundamental questions of lack of respect for the human personality as such. This lack of respect is endemic in society as a whole, but it particularly grates with me in the case of psychiatry, as the latter is supposed by the layman to have the purpose of alleviating mental distress.

It is not just a question of things being done badly, rather than well. It is more a question of whether certain things should be done at all, and whether things should be looked at in one way, rather than another. This book will deal with these questions, and will conclude by questioning the validity of the profession of psychiatry as such.

This book is very much indebted to the writings of Thomas Szasz, Peter Breggin, and Lucy Johnstone in particular, and to conversations with Pamela Jenkinson. I am also indebted to Leonard Roy Frank and Ronald Bassman, among others, for their accounts of their personal experiences. With regard to psychoanalysis, I am very much indebted to George Frankl for his account of his methods in his two books, "*The Unknown Self*" and "*Exploring The Unconscious*", and also for the help he gave me as my analyst for many years. I would also like to acknowledge the encouragement of Sheila Camino in recent years. However, the general thrust of the book and its conclusions are my own.

I would like to stress that my hostility to psychiatrists in this book is a hostility to those psychiatrists who are rigid adherents of the medical model and do not acknowledge their patients as real human beings. It is not directed at those psychiatrists who treat their patients in a humane way and try to help them.

1

Actual Diseases Of The Brain And Nervous System

There are a number of conditions of organic origin and cases of brain injuries, with severely damaging affects on mental processes and behaviour. These must be sharply distinguished from the conditions termed 'mental illnesses'. At one time, all these conditions were lumped together, but the advance in medical knowledge has enabled the two categories to be separated.

In the former cases, there are definite tests, similar to those used in the rest of medicine, to determine whether a person has the damaging condition or not. In the case of Alzheimer's disease, the fact that somebody had the disease can be definitely determined by a post-mortem examination of the brain, although brain scans while the person is alive do not necessarily give a clear result. Parkinson's disease definitely affects a particular part of the brain. There is a definite scientific reason for the application of drugs such as L-Dopa to alleviate, and perhaps slow down, the progress of Parkinson's. In the case of Alzheimer's, there is at present no drug which will do any good, but it may be that such a drug will be available in the near future. In both cases, the injection of brain cells is thought of as a possible remedy in the future. Such a treatment would presumably enhance brain-power, and prevent brain deterioration.

What is not in doubt, in the cases of Alzheimer's and Parkinson's, is the physical basis of both of these conditions. This is true, not just in the trivial sense that everything mental has something in the brain related to it, but that the state of the brain in both cases is not normal.

Another aspect of these two conditions is that people can succumb to them, regardless of any previous behaviour or state of mind which they might have. There is nothing mental about these afflictions, though the behaviour of the person (and, in the case of Alzheimer's, their state of mind and mental activity) will be severely debilitated.

Epilepsy is another condition with a definite physical base. In fact, there are a number of different types of Epilepsy. The Epileptic seizure, when it occurs, is an obvious physical phenomenon. Detection is generally done by brain scans, Electroencephalography (EEG) or Magnetic Resonance Imaging (MRI). For prevention or alleviation of the seizures, various anti-epileptic drugs are used. These do have undesirable side affects, and the advantages have to be balanced against this. However, here again, there is no question of anything mental having anything to do with the condition, though there are several possible causes of it.

Strokes, brain tumours, and brain damage from external causes have affects on both mental and physical capacities of individuals, and sometimes on their behaviour. In these situations, the physical cause of the mental or physical damage is obvious.

In all these cases, the damage has been caused by physical conditions. The moral dictated by the situation is not to make the damage worse. Sometimes brain operations are performed, but the improvement expected from the operation should never be at the expense of any loss of vital mental function.

With regard to the loss of mental function in any respect and from whatever cause, the writings of Oliver Sacks are extremely relevant. In his writings, he shows that however debilitated the condition of the patient is, he still treats him or her as a human being, and recognises what capacity the patient still possesses, as well as what he or she has lost. In this, he shows himself as a physician possessing moral qualities in addition to scientific expertise.

In these situations of actual brain diseases or of damage to the brain or nervous system, the organic nature of the disease or damage can be detected by a pathologist in autopsies after the person is dead. In contrast, in the case of schizophrenia or other mental illnesses diagnosed by psychiatrists, there is no pathological test, though the affects of damaging psychiatric treatments on the brain may be evident.

In the case of what are called mental illnesses, no organic basis of them has been found. Therefore, there are no grounds for the physical and medical treatments prescribed by the psychiatrists. But even if an organic basis was found in the future, which I strongly predict will not happen, any treatment acceptable to ethically-minded people would not involve the infliction of brain damage in addition to the mental illness which the patient was deemed to be suffering from. An acceptable treatment would have to target the alleged mental illness, and leave every other aspect of the mind and the personality intact. The physical and medical treatments prescribed by the psychiatrists do not target the alleged illness, but affect every aspect of the mind. I do not believe that what are called mental illnesses can be put under the same classification as medical illnesses, but, even if they could be, the treatments producing brain damage are completely unacceptable.

From time to time, people will say that the cause of this or that physical illness was psychosomatic, and often this may well be true, though it could never be proved. But this would not provide any more work for the psychiatrists, since their treatments are not psychological but medical. It would give work to psychotherapists, provided the psychosomatic aspect was suspected in time. Of course, psychotherapy in these cases would not always be successful, but it would be worth a try. However, this whole subject is outside the scope of this book. I mention it merely in passing.

2

The Unknown Soldier At
The Cenotaph

We are all familiar with the tomb of The Unknown Soldier at the Cenotaph in Whitehall in London. We know that the body of a soldier was taken at random from the dead on the battlefields of the 1st World War, and brought to London to be reburied at the Cenotaph. His name was unknown to us, because he was meant to represent all those who had died for their country in the war. Being unknown, he could be anyone of those who had died. That was right and proper. It expressed the acknowledgement of the sacrifice of the soldiers by the country for which they had fought.

Supposing we knew that his actual name was Joe Bloggs. Would he now be known to us, or would he still be unknown? For the particular purpose of his burial at the Cenotaph, he would now be known, and this fact would present a problem. But, in a more profound sense, he would still be unknown.

If we contacted all those who had known Joe Bloggs in his life, his family, friends, and associates, could they be said to really know Joe Bloggs? They would know a number of things about him, but the answer is no. And supposing Joe Bloggs had experienced mental problems and had consulted a psychotherapist, could he or she be said to really know Joe Bloggs? The answer again is no, although he or she might also know a number of things about him. But, throughout his life, Joe Bloggs knew things about himself which nobody else knew.

We may wish to know the thoughts and feelings of Joe Bloggs. He need not tell us what they are. We may think that he had a certain character. We may be right. But Joe Bloggs had his own motivations. And they may not coincide with ours. He may dislike us. That does not matter. We may dislike him. That does not matter, either. Our respect for him is because he, like ourselves, is part of humanity. The unique personality of each human being, which is in a profound sense unknown to us, demands our acknowledgement and respect.

3

A Personal Experience

Decisions to become involved in a particular cause often have their origins in some personal experience, and that is the case with me in writing this book.

In my early twenties, having completed a university degree and after working in a solicitor's office for a time, and not liking it, I went to work in a library as a temporary measure. Having not learnt the piano as a child, I suddenly decided that I wanted to learn to play it as an adult. My piano teacher, a very gifted person, was in the process of becoming a concert pianist.

I worked hard at the piano and, not having a natural talent, found the necessary coordination difficult. However, I developed a friendship with my teacher. After a time, she mentioned to me that she had a friend whom she would like me to meet. A meeting was arranged, and the friend was in fact a psychoanalyst. My piano teacher was very sensitive, and she had realised that I was not making the best of myself, and was in fact a very repressed individual.

So began the long period of psychoanalysis that culminated in my becoming the relatively confident and contented person that I am today. I was willing to embark on psychoanalysis, since I had felt for some time that all was not well with me. I had a stammer, and had been to a speech therapist, but that was just dealing with a symptom. I had also been to somebody who gave helpful advice about careers. But I did not just want someone to help me to adjust to the person I appeared to be. I wanted someone who would help me to release the real person

I instinctively felt I was, instead of the repressed personality I was at the time.

My psychoanalysis started off with sessions of twice a week and then once a week, and then it was reduced to longer and longer periods between sessions. In the closing years of my association with my analyst, I just went to see him very occasionally as a friend.

He said to me once that some orthodox analysts favoured a totally non-interactive approach. With the patient lying on the couch they stayed absolutely mute while he or she poured forth whatever came into their minds. My analyst was much more human than that, and talked normally with his patients. In spite of having experienced a full share of adversity in his life, he was quite a cheerful person. I became great friends with him, and felt that I could talk to him about anything. That was the case with most of his patients. He was not a person remote from the world. There were things he felt strongly about and he showed it. I remember at the time of the Six Day War, he was overjoyed at the Israeli victory. Occasionally, he talked of his childhood and of his brother. I respected him for all this. It made him more human.

As my psychoanalysis progressed, a considerable amount of things emerged from my unconscious together with their attendant emotions. This comprised mostly tremendous fears and tremendous anger, which I had repressed under a veneer of cold and unemotional respectability. Even my mother said that I had gone into a shell. My fears had prevented me from entering any situation where I would be likely to have to face them. This was very restrictive of my life, as well as making me very ashamed of myself. And the repressed anger made my relations with other people difficult.

My analyst not only helped me to gain access to things which I had buried in my unconscious, together with their accompanying emotions. He also gave me some guidance and encouragement in my daily life, and in the decisions about my career. Altogether, things gradually improved for me, and I am very grateful to him.

Sometimes I got impatient, and wanted to make changes in my life before he considered I was ready for them. But I think, in retrospect, that he was right. The consequences of a move in the right direction before I was ready for it could have been counterproductive. And if, at times, I failed to follow my own initiatives, the fault lay with me, and not with him. You cannot expect a therapist to do everything for you. You have to do things for yourself. And this becomes even more the case as the therapy advances, and you grow stronger.

I said that, at the beginning of my analysis, I had a lot of repressed anger. When this came to the surface in the therapy, some of this anger was against my family. But I was living by myself, and not with my family at the time, so there were only very rare occasions when I expressed overt anger against them. However, with the help of my analyst, I managed to keep things in proportion, and I came to realise that things were not that simple, and that they were only partly to blame, and also that they had had their own troubles. After a short time, my relations with my family became reasonably cordial. In fact, they became better than they had been before, since the shell I had wrapped around myself had become much thinner.

Some people, in reading this account, might conclude that I had not had a really serious mental illness. If by a serious mental illness is meant a psychosis, then that is true, but I did have a neurosis. Throughout my darkest period, I was still living in a fairly protected environment, and did not have any severe irritants from the outside world impinging on me. If I had not been living in this fairly protected environment, my mental state would probably have been much worse.

Two things worked to my advantage. The first is that throughout my life, both before and during the period of my analysis, I never really lost control. I had lost my temper on occasions, but losing control is a longer-lasting and much more complete experience. I have always been very afraid of losing

control, and I never have. I have never had a feeling of
complete helplessness. The second is that I have always been
in the very fortunate position of having a private income. It
has not made me rich, and I have always been relatively frugal.
But I have never been entirely dependant on what I earned. It
has meant that I have had a greater degree of freedom than
those without it. Of course, if I had married and had children
I would have lost much of this freedom. But I never did. The
reason is this. I am a heterosexual with normal feelings. But I
have never found a girl with whom I felt sufficient affinity to
take this step. And I did not want to marry and have children
just for the sake of it. I realised instinctively that that could
have ended in disaster.

When I look back on my life and on my mental troubles
from the vantage point of the person I am now, my reflections
are quite interesting. Some people might have regrets. They
might think that they could have lived more conventional and
enjoyable lives. They might think that they could have had
worldly success. They might think that they could have had
happy marriages and happy family lives. They could have
done things differently. In fact, they could have been different
persons altogether. For that is the logical conclusion to this
way of thinking.

There is some good in the person I am now, and there is
some good in the life I have experienced. For if I had not had
these mental troubles, and if I had not had my particular
personality, I would not be the person I am now. I pride myself
on having a certain insight into psychological matters, and into
public affairs. I have an ability to think outside the box. But
where do I get this insight and this ability from? It can only be
from having had my mental troubles, and from not having had
a life of conventional success.

You are the person you are, and there is a limit to how much
you can change your life without becoming a totally different
individual. You can strive to improve yourself, but you cannot
change yourself entirely. And the concentration on regrets is a

desire to do this. If you understand this, the experience of mental troubles can make a positive contribution to the formation of character and personality.

The story with a happy ending which I have just related would not have been possible if I had not been able to pay for private psychoanalysis. Also, if my piano teacher had not put me in touch with my analyst. I have gradually come to realise how terrible my situation could have been if I had had to rely on the state's psychiatric services. I therefore, feel a debt of gratitude for my good fortune and a determination to end the debilitating treatments given out to my fellow human beings.

4

The Beginnings Of Psychiatry

P sychiatry as a profession had its beginnings in the 19th century.

A great many of those who would later be designated as mad remained in the community. Some of those dependant on the parish for their upkeep were put into institutions such as Bedlam. There were also a great number of private institutions, mostly containing small numbers of inmates, which were run for profit by private individuals. These were sometimes clergymen, sometimes doctors, and often just ordinary people who chose to do this. The inmates in these institutions were often treated very badly, and they were frequently put in chains. However, in some places catering for the wealthiest members of society, the inmates lived a life similar to that of their own homes, save for the fact that they were deprived of their liberty.

In the early years of the 19th century, there arose a movement with a different philosophy of treatment for the insane. This was the philosophy of "moral treatment". It originated with the the Quakers, and is associated with the name of Samuel Tuke and his institution called the York Retreat. It did not believe in coercion of any kind, but thought that the insane were best dealt with by kindness and sympathy and wholesome occupations.

The Tukes were not doctors. Nor were the other people engaged in running the York Retreat and similar places. They thought that medicine had nothing to offer in this field. When doctors had tried their various remedies such as bleeding, blisters, electric shocks, cold baths, and drugs of various kinds, the results had not been encouraging. But the Tukes believed that non-medical people were as suitable for caring for the insane as medical people, and the methods of the Tukes had considerable success.

The medical profession did not like this. They wanted to be the acknowledged experts in this field and made every effort to convince the public to let them establish a monopoly. This eventually happened, with every county being required by law to build asylums for the insane to be run by qualified doctors.

This was not inevitable, and it was not in the interests of the inmates. Of course, the old disorganised system where there was no proper regulation of the treatment given needed to be improved. But to build big asylums for great numbers of inmates, rather than small ones for far fewer, was a big mistake. And to insist on medical personnel being in charge was another big mistake.

The trouble was that the protagonists of "moral treatment" sounded as if they were in favour of something a bit nebulous. In actual fact, the success rate of "moral treatment", with respect to the number of people getting better, was far in excess of anything achieved by the doctors. But the doctors could talk in semi-scientific language, and they were supported by medical journals which could do the same. The protagonists of "moral treatment" were up against a very formidable opponent, and they needed to mount a propaganda campaign as intense as the latter.

There was another factor which swayed many of the public in favour of the doctors, and that was that the distress in which people with mental problems usually were seemed to resemble at least superficially the distress in people with genuine illnesses. The ordinary person tended to link distress and illness together, thus favouring the doctors.

The protagonists of "moral treatment", unlike the doctors, had not organised themselves into a profession. So the doctors were put in charge of the new asylums, and were regarded as the proper people to be consulted about "mental" matters. Thus the psychiatric profession was born. The doctors in these new asylums had nothing to offer of a medical nature to the inmates, though later they would try to do so. They were in fact custodians, and the inmates were their captives. But this did not worry their real clients, the relatives of the patients and the parish councils that were paying the bills. Whether a treatment was more likely to produce an improvement in the patient was a secondary consideration to these people. Basically they were grateful to anybody who would take the care of these unwanted people off their hands. Whether the semi-scientific defences of psychiatric activities made any sense to the ostensible patients was not important.

For some time, the doctors or psychiatrists, as they came to be called, were just custodians. But this did not content them. They thought of themselves as doctors, and they wished to offer some kind of medical treatment, whether genuine or not. In general, there was nothing physically wrong with the inmates, though their behaviour was often weird. So the psychiatrists classified the various weird behaviours of the inmates with the names of impressive-sounding mental illnesses, and persuaded themselves that there was an organic cause for each of the various conditions. The fact that they did not find an organic cause did not deter them. They acted as if the organic cause had been discovered, or was about to be discovered very soon, and they have continued along the same line ever since. The psychiatrists treated these people with medical treatments as if they were dealing with genuine medical ailments, even though there was no proven connection between what they were suffering from and the treatments. They also continually tried to expand their empire by diagnosing more and more behaviour as signs of mental illness.

All this was possible for three reasons:-
   1) The concept of mental illness was, and is, exceptionally vague. There were no objective tests for it.

2) Anybody regarded as mad was, and is, thought of as outside civilised society and its norms.

3) The real people who had to be satisfied with the situation were not the inmates of the asylums, but the local authorities and the relatives.

5

Madness

Madness was, and is, regarded as a condition apart from that of the general run of humanity. Mad people were, and still are to a large extent, regarded as significantly different from normal people. At one time, they comprised everybody whose behaviour appeared as not normal, whatever the cause of their condition. So the mentally defective, those who had developed brain diseases, and those suffering from what are now designated as mental illnesses, were all lumped together, and were confined in various institutions, large or small, set aside for them. Sometimes people whose behaviour offended against the prevailing norms, such as unmarried mothers, were also confined.

People designated as mad tended to behave in strange and unconventional ways. They could be difficult to deal with, and their family or relatives felt that to have these people living with them would interfere with their own lives and their social intercourse with people at large. They wanted the people designated as mad out of the way.

Madness was behaviour beyond the realms of normal understanding. People were afraid of it. The last thing they wanted was any hint that there could be anything strange in their own behaviour. There must be a firm line in the sand: on one side were the mad people, and on the other side were the sane people like themselves. These attitudes, though in reduced intensity, are very prevalent today.

Another important aspect of madness is this. No credibility was, and is, given to what those designated as mad say.

Whatever they say is said to be an aspect of their madness. They are in a very dangerous situation. Their situation is worse than that of criminals who have offended against the laws of the land. The latter have acknowledged rights. They can be protected by solicitors, and what they say is responded to in a normal fashion, since they are assumed to be rational. But those thought of as mad are not considered rational. Therefore, everybody who has anything to do with them accepts this, unless they choose to dispute it. It derives from the designation of them as mad given to them by psychiatrists.

The fact that what they say is ignored has had dire consequences for those designated as mad. It has meant that they have had no say as to the treatment they receive, and it has meant that their relationships with family and friends and their status in the outside world are also adversely affected.

6

Physical And Chemical Treatments

Lobotomy and ECT

Among all the various physical treatments of one kind or another to which psychiatrists have subjected the inmates in their care, some have been particularly horrendous. The most horrendous were the lobotomies performed on the helpless inmates. The operation of pre-frontal lobotomy was first performed by Egas Moniz, and subsequently by such people as Walter Freeman in America, and others in Britain. It was hailed by much of the psychiatric establishment as a psychiatric breakthrough for dealing with cases not responsive to other treatments. In actual fact, the lobotomies were synonymous with brain damage. They involve the destruction of healthy brain tissue. This goes dead against the taboo against destroying or damaging healthy bodily organs that is the rule in ordinary medicine.

One of the most horrendous lobotomies was that performed on Rosemary Kennedy, the elder daughter of Joseph Kennedy and sister of President Kennedy. Her fault in the eyes of her father was probably that she was a bit simple, and might disgrace the family. So he took her to Walter Freeman, who performed a lobotomy on her. This transformed her into a complete vegetable with childlike behaviour. This shows that the culprits in this appalling business were not only the psychiatrists involved, but could also be relatives. Though the results of the operation were not always as severe as in this case, it has almost always been said of a person subjected to a lobotomy that they were not the same person afterwards,and that their original personality had been destroyed. In my opinion,to perform a lobotomy on someone is worse than killing them, and anybody who performs this operation is beyond the pale. No condition of the patient can possibly justify it.

Another treatment producing brain damage is Electroconvulsive Shock Treatment (ECT). This is not as horrific as lobotomy, but it can still be severely damaging. The first performance of ECT on a patient was by Ugo Cerletti in Italy, just before the 2nd World War. ECT produces a convulsion by passing an electric current through the brain, but a similar effect had been produced by Insulin Coma Therapy. Like lobotomy, the treatment of ECT was purely experimental. There was no serious insight into the illness supposed to be cured by it. The psychiatrists experimented to see what was the result.

ECT always causes a certain amount of loss of memory. Sometimes this results in the loss of acquired skills. There was a case of a concert pianist who lost her memory of her entire concert repertoire. Another person who,before receiving ECT, was very good at mathematics,found that,after treatment with ECT, he was just average. Often a person's memory of treasured events in their life is lost, forcing them to ask relatives to fill in the gaps. Of course,even when a relative does remind the person of the past event, that does not give back to the person the emotions that the past event originally evoked. There was the famous case of Ernest Hemmingway who,after receiving ECT said that it effectively destroyed his ability to write, since that was dependent on his memory being intact. He therefore committed suicide. The damage is not always as great as in these cases, but there is always some damage.

There is the comment on ECT by Sidney Samant MD in the American journal, *Clinical Psychiatry News*, for March 1983: "As a neurologist and electro-encephalographer, I have seen many patients after ECT, and I have no doubt that ECT produces effects identical to those of a head injury. After multiple sessions of ECT, a patient has symptoms identical to those of a retired, punch-drunk boxer. After a few sessions of ECT the symptoms are those of a moderate cerebral contusion, and further enthusiastic use of ECT may result in the patient functioning at a subhuman level. ECT may be defined as a controlled type of brain damage produced by electrical means."

In some cases of ECT treatment, the damage can be compared to the loss of a limb, or the deterioration of one of the person's faculties.

Sometimes people who have received ECT (or even in some rare cases some who have had a lobotomy) may, after great struggle, make something of their lives, and do well. Such a person is Leonard Roy Frank, a survivor of ECT, and a campaigner against it. But the successes of these people testify to the indomitability of the human spirit against the odds, and not to any alleged benefit of the treatment.

Some psychiatrists who have performed lobotomies or ECT have in a moment of candour admitted the truth about these operations. They have said that it is the brain damage that produces the cure, or that some people have too much brain. Of course, when you experience brain damage of this magnitude, your mental problems will be dampened along with the rest of you. But people who say these things reveal themselves as the enemies of everything that makes us human. People like that should never be allowed anywhere near medicine or the caring professions.

Treatment with drugs

It is very much the rule for psychiatrists, unless they are also psychotherapists, to treat their patients with drugs. There are the neuroleptics, the antidepressants, and the minor tranquilizers. Of these, there are a number of different brands, each proclaimed to be the wonder drug by its manufacturer and the psychiatrists who prescribe them.

Usually, these drugs are taken over a considerable period of time. The affect of taking a single dose, though unpleasant and making a person feel spaced-out, would not be disastrous. One friend of mine had financial and health worries, and was prescribed a psychiatric drug because he was depressed about this. He felt awful, and definitely not his usual self. So he stopped taking them after a few doses. However, taken regularly over a period of time there may be considerably more adverse affects. These may be tardive dyskinesia, with its permanent untreatable tics and spasms of the voluntary muscles. Another friend of mine had his sex life ruined through prolonged taking of drugs for his panic attacks. There may even be tardive dementia, with its permanent deterioration of mental capacity. There can even be reduction in the size of a person's brain (revealed in an autopsy after death) through taking these drugs. At the very least, the person will be operating at a reduced level in every way while he or she is taking them. Many psychiatric drugs are highly addictive. If a person tries to come off one of these drugs suddenly, they may suffer severe withdrawal symptoms. However, it is possible to come off them gradually with a bit of emotional support. A further danger of psychiatric drugs was brought to my attention recently. The father of a friend of mine had been taking psychiatric drugs for a number of years. He has recently been diagnosed with Alzheimer's disease. There is no proof that there is a connection between the two, but many of us will suspect that there is.

Peter Breggin writes that, instead of treating a disease, the neuroleptic drugs create a disease. Delay and Deniker were the first psychiatrists to experiment with Thorazine. They immediately noticed that small doses produced a neurological disease very similar to a special type of virulent flu, called lethargic encephalitis, that killed tens of thousands during and shortly after the 1st World War. And encephalitis means inflamation of the brain. There is no mention of this important information in the psychiatric literature, so that most young psychiatrists are not aware of it. Both viral encephalitis and drug-induced neuroleptic malignant syndrome are marked by lobotomy-like indifference, which progress to fever and sweating, unstable cardiovascular signs, bizarre dyskinesias, and in severe cases, delirium, coma, and death. Meanwhile, there can be permanent parkinsonism, and psychotic states, or dementia.

From the point of view of the psychiatrist, the prescription of drugs does not take up too much time, and does not require any great communication with or rapport with the patient. Another boon is that drugged patients are easier to manage. This is particularly helpful to the psychiatrists in institutions such as mental asylums. In the past, patients in mental institutions were put in straight-jackets, allegedly to stop them harming themselves. Now they are given drugs which act as chemical straight-jackets. Personally, I would prefer the original straight jackets. At least my brain would be intact. But the drugs have the advantage, for some people, of being invisible. Everything is supposed to be all right, as long as the force used is disguised, and does not stare you in the face.

Another beneficiary of the prescription of psychiatric drugs is the pharmaceutical industry which manufactures them. It may be wondered what kind of testing is required for putting these drugs on the market. In fact, a drug is generally approved if it dampens the patient in the required way, with any ill-affects mentioned, if at all, as side affects. Extreme affects of the drugs are not usually clearly advertised, as that would reduce the enthusiasm for them.

Of course, the patient's so-called mental illness will be diminished in its emotional intensity by the action of the drugs, along with the rest of his or her intellectual, physical, and emotional life. The same is true of ECT and lobotomy as psychiatric treatments. This supports the claim that these treatments produce cures in the short term. In the long term, it is a different story. But the public are not told about this. The official version is that psychiatric drugs and ECT target the particular mental illness for which the patient has been diagnosed, supposedly leaving everything else more-or-less intact. This is not so.

Psychiatric and Recreational Drugs

Recreational drugs such as LSD and Cannabis come under official condemnation, and alcohol and tobacco are definitely disapproved of. With regard to alcohol, excessive drinking of it is condemned, and the medical establishment disapproves of alcoholics. The dangers to health and to mental and physical activity are pointed out. The addictive qualities of alcohol are also understood. Alcoholism has even a psychiatric classification as a mental illness. Smoking,too,has been condemned by the medical establishment, and has been banned in public places. With regard to LSD and Cannabis, these are classified as illegal substances, and it is against the law to imbibe these drugs,and still more to sell them. The medical establishment points out the dangers of brain damage through taking these drugs.

It is interesting that all the above substances are things which people desire to take. They give the person taking them a good feeling. Nevertheless, they are harmful. People are stupid to start taking them. In the case of LSD and Cannabis, they have sometimes wrecked peoples' lives. And the medical establishment is right in its condemnations, and the Government is right in the measures which it has taken.

But there is hypocrisy on the part of both the medical establishment and the Government. For their attitude to psychiatric drugs, if prescribed by qualified psychiatrists, is one of approval. Yet they, too, can be dangerous. They, too, can be addictive. They, too, can wreck peoples' lives. The only difference is that mostly nobody wants to take them.

The real difference between the two sets of drugs is that one set carries the seal of approval of authority with the proclaimed fiction that they can cure people of ailments, while the other set does not. In fact, the recreational drugs are taken in defiance of authority. Could it be the case that the medical establishment and the government are less concerned about the actual welfare of the consumers of drugs than about whether their authority is being defied or complied with?

The Real Truth About Drugs

In this section I am heavily indebted to the views of Joanna Moncrieff as expressed in her book, "*Psychiatric Drugs*". The present thinking of the psychiatric establishment is that psychiatric drugs target and cure distinct mental illnesses. The view is that mental illnesses are biologically caused. The drugs are supposed to counteract various supposed abnormalities of the brain. This is the disease-centred model of the action of psychiatric drugs. In actual fact, no such abnormalities have been proved to exist in the brains of mentally disturbed people. Indeed, if any abnormalities are observed, they are the result of the actions of the psychiatric drugs. The disease-centred model is part-and-parcel of the desire of the psychiatric establishment that psychiatry should be recognised as just another speciality of orthodox medicine, and that it should be medical in the remedies it provides.

There is another way of looking at the action of psychiatric drugs, and that is the drug-centred model. This treats psychiatric drugs like any other drugs, it denies that any of them target any particular mental illness, and concentrates on what particular drugs actually do. The dangers of brain damage or Parkinson-type affects or the dangers to physical and mental health in general through the taking of any particular drug in the short term or the long term are noted. The advantages, if any, of using the drugs as sedatives for severely disturbed people, balanced against the dangers, are noted. In deciding to use any of the drugs in this way, the recipient has to be fully aware of the dangers as well as any advantages, and if he or she is a minor, then the parent or guardian would need to be fully aware. Provided the dangers are understood, it can be helpful for a person in the most intense period of depression to take anti-depressants to tide them over this period. This was pointed out by Dorothy Rowe in her book, "*Depression*", on pages 222 and 223. The advantage is that the drugs help to distance the person from the distressing thoughts, and so give the person some psychic space, but the drugs do not make the distressing thoughts disappear. For dealing with that, psychotherapy or psycho-analysis is needed. This is plainly a use of drugs according to the drug-centred model, and not the disease-centred model.

Since the disease-centred model is the orthodox view, the targeting of a particular mental illness by a particular drug is accepted by many people without question. It is not realised that the research supporting this is partial and misleading. In short, anything which can be produced to support the orthodox view is brought forward, whereas anything which does not support it is ignored. When a particular drug is tested for its efficacy with a group who receive it against a control group who receive placebos, the test is the percentage who are well enough to leave the hospital or asylum without returning. But the test period is always relatively short. If somebody decides to come off any particular drug, there is usually an adverse reaction due to withdrawal symptoms. This fact is taken advantage of by the pro-drug lobby to say that continuing to take the drug prevents a recurrence of the mental illness. But it is the presence of withdrawal symptoms that is the problem, and not the mental illness. All this means is that people should come off the drug gradually. Further, whatever damage is caused by the drugs is falsely stated to be due to the underlying mental illness, whereas really the damage is caused by the drugs.

In short, the disease-centred model of the action of psychiatric drugs as well as the disease-centred model of mental illnesses are unproven, and are motivated by the desire of its supporters to see things from the biopsychiatric viewpoint. The drug-centred model, on the other hand, is concerned with reality.

7

Psychiatric Diagnosis
And Symptoms

Underlying the practise of orthodox psychiatry are the various classifications which have been given to the types of behaviour considered as symptomatic of mental illness. The two main types of the more serious disorders, known as psychoses, are schizophrenia and manic depression, also known as bipolar disorder, and there are also sub-classifications of these. In addition, there are the neuroses, which are less serious.

To be diagnosed as suffering from schizophrenia, or manic depression, or any of the other disorders, the person diagnosed must display certain symptoms over a period of time. The symptoms which are species of behaviour are the only tests. There are no physical tests as there are in general medicine. The tests are therefore subjective, and psychiatrists may disagree about which classification the prospective patient's symptoms fall under. For instance, people are much more frequently diagnosed with schizophrenia, as opposed to the other classifications, in America than in Britain. Many people may have the symptoms of both schizophrenia and manic depression. The idea that mental illness can be divided into several neat categories of disorder in the same way that bodily illness can is an illusion.

Further, many of the symptoms of schizophrenia or manic depression are characteristic of people who do not regard themselves as having a mental illness. There are auditory hallucinations, the hearing of voices which are not there. Many people throughout the ages have experienced these, just as some people have experienced visual hallucinations. Then there are the delusions of grandeur, the thinking that you are Napoleon, or Christ, or someone important. Now, all sorts of people think many strange things without regarding themselves as mentally ill, and without others regarding them in this way either, and some of these people can be very obsessive and obstinate in their beliefs. Very often, people who are said to be mentally ill have complexes of being persecuted. Many people feel this way at certain times of their lives. Such things as deterioration from a previous level of functioning in such areas as work, social relations, and self-care, count as symptoms. Under this heading is a marked impairment in personal hygiene or grooming. Social isolation or withdrawal from society also count as symptoms. Indeed, if one goes through all the (Diagnostic and Statistical Manual of Mental Disorders (DSM) DSM-111 criteria for inferring schizophrenia, all of them are symptoms that most people experience when they are in particular moods at various times of their lives. If we are not careful, a considerable proportion of the population could be diagnosed by the psychiatrists as mentally ill.

These symptoms, from which psychiatrists infer the existence of mental illnesses, can be explained in terms of the person's life experiences. People do not show such symptoms for no reason. And the reason is not a mysterious biological illness, but a reaction to childhood experiences, or to events which occurred in the person's life.

Politics has also been involved in psychiatric classifications.

Before the American Civil War, when slavery was legal in the Southern states, there was a psychiatric diagnosis called drapetomania found among the Negro slaves, which was the urge to escape from slavery. It was not sufficient for the owners to endeavour to prevent them escaping. In addition, they diagnosed them as mad for wanting to do so.

Throughout the 19th and well into the 20th centuries, the practise of masturbation both among men and women and young and old was thought of by a great many doctors and psychiatrists as liable to give rise to insanity. This gave rise to some of them resorting to some very unpleasant measures to curtail it.

For a long time, homosexuality was diagnosed as a mental illness, and psychiatrists tried by various methods to transform homosexuals into heterosexuals. It has only been pressure from the gay community and public opinion at large which has caused this to be reversed.

In the cases of masturbation and homosexuality, the condemnations from the psychiatrists followed the condemnations from religious bodies. In fact, religious strictures were transformed into medical strictures.

The particular designation known as Masochistic Personality Disorder was withdrawn, owing to pressure from the feminist lobby.

For a long time, epilepsy was treated as a psychiatric illness, and epileptics were treated with the same sort of constraints as other psychiatric patients. But as soon as it was diagnosed as a definite neurological condition, epileptics were allowed to lead normal lives, apart from the requirement to take pills to prevent epileptic fits.

ADHD

Attention Deficit Hyperactivity Disorder (ADHD) for short, is a recent psychiatric classification applied to children and teenagers. Fred Baughman in his book, *"The ADHD Fraud"*, explains how psychiatry makes patients out of normal children. He describes what is happening in America, but the same thing is showing signs of happening in this country too.

The ADHD classification is most often applied to the normal high-spirited behaviour of young people. The classification is brought forward when adults find children or young people difficult to handle. The background behind this may be uninspiring teaching at school or a bad environment at home, for neither of which is the youngster responsible.

The result of an ADHD classification being applied by the psychiatrist is that the youngster is compulsorarily drugged, with all the dangers for him or her which that implies, and in addition the ADHD classification remains on his or her medical records. There was a very tragic case recently, when a ten-year-old boy hanged himself after being put on a dose of the drug Ritalin for a number of years. These drugs do irreparable damage. The ADHD classification is applied to normal kids, whom the adults cannot control.

This is a flagrant example of biopsychiatric imperialism. Instead of the real problems of the youngsters being attended to, they are drugged. This lets off the hook inadequate teachers or inadequate parents. Of course, the psychiatrists will earn a lot of money, and so will the drug companies.

There is another aspect of this, and that is the decline of the traditional ways of disciplining children and young people. There is no doubt that some youngsters are troublesome and sometimes violent. The traditional methods of discipline coped with this. They may have been disliked by the youngsters and sometimes by the parents, but there was nothing underhand about them. They did not cause brain damage, and the long term prospects for the youngsters were not impaired. It may be that the abolition of ADHD with its drugging of youngsters would be helped by a return to the traditional methods of discipline and communication.

This is a very serious subject. We have here the threat of brain damage to a sizeable part of the young people of this country. For all our sakes, it must combated with the utmost vigour.

The real trouble with psychiatric classifications is the use to which they have been put. They are thought of as similar to medical classifications, and they are used to support the giving of pseudo-medical treatment to psychiatric patients. They are also the basis of the power of the psychiatrists to section people, and the presence of a psychiatric classification on someone's medical records can stand against that person in job applications. In fact, the original decision to apply a certain psychiatric label to a certain group of patients was no great discovery. It was simply an example of the universal habit of describing people in certain ways to make life less chaotic. Psychoanalysts and psychotherapists can, if they so choose, use these classifications. But with them it is just the start in a investigation into what is behind the mental distress of the client, and a commencement of therapy to relieve that distress. With psychiatrists, it is the start of arbitrary pseudo-medical treatment.

8

The Real Situation

What are called mental illnesses do not belong in the sphere of medicine at all. They belong to the sphere of the rest of life. Only if an illness has been proven to have a medical cause can it be said to be an illness. Mental illnesses have never been proved to have this. And if what has hitherto been called a mental illness were to be proved to have a medical cause, then it would become the proper subject of study for the neurologist, not the psychiatrist. This is not to deny that a person with mental troubles can be in very great distress, so severe that he or she could be considered ill. But people who have experienced great sorrow are also in very great distress.

With mental illnesses, it is a case of the mind affecting both body and mind, rather than the body affecting the mind.

Dorothy Rowe, in her book *"Beyond Fear"*, discusses how various mental illnesses such as Anxiety and Phobias, Obsessions and Compulsions, Depression, Mania, and Schizophrenia arise. She also gives a good description of the fantasy world of a person who could be considered as schizophrenic. She described it as making sense in view of the psychic background of the person.

Mental illnesses can be distinguished from genuine brain diseases or brain injuries. A person who suffers from the latter has a diminished capacity. The person who suffers from what is termed a mental illness has needed to be clever enough to have the mental illness. The symptoms of the two are different.

A person with a brain disease or brain injury would not be able to have hallucinations or elaborate *follies de grandeur*. Human beings are very clever. They are clever enough to tie themselves in knots. Of course, the person suffering from what is called a mental illness is also handicapped, but it is a handicap which the person has chosen to have. He or she has chosen to suffer from this handicap as a way of dealing with some traumas or misfortunes which have been experienced in the past. We can compare this situation to that of someone at a road junction with a choice of two directions in which to go. If he takes the road which he would normally take, and which would bring him to his final destination, he will encounter a ferocious beast, which will do him great harm. If he takes the other road he may not reach his final destination, but he will avoid the beast, and this is what he chooses to do.

In some ways, the workings of computers present a situation analogous to that of human beings. With computers, there is the hardware and the software. Most of the time, if you have problems with your computer, it is a problem to do with the software. It is very rare that your problem is to do with the hardware. And no-one would dream of dealing with a software problem by fiddling about with the hardware. But this is what the biopsychiatrists are doing all the time, when they fiddle about with the brain when somebody has mental troubles.

A very great part of our lives is social. Even when we are alone, our relations with our fellow human beings have importance for us. Just as important as the sexual attraction between people is the rivalry between them and the desire of each to win the acclamation of his or her fellows. There are two great motivating factors in human beings, the love for those we love, and the desire for self preservation accomplished by using our intelligence, strength, and cunning. Although some of the feelings and emotions which we have during our lives are due to physical illnesses and accidents, the majority of them are due to our interactions with other people.

The intervention of the psychiatric establishment in this maelstrom of human relationships can often be likened to that of a bull in a china shop, who decides to batter an already broken piece of crockery. The intervention of a psychotherapist in the maelstrom is totally different. A good psychotherapist understands the maelstrom of human relationships, and can therefore make a valid contribution. But treatments such as drugs and ECT do not relate at all, but just suppress the already vulnerable individual. The psychiatrist who uses these treatments is not neutral politically, but is acting as the ally of all those who have succeeded in suppressing the individual in the past.

The Two Worlds

Let us imagine reality as consisting of two worlds, the world of science, and our world. Accompanying us on our visit to the world of science will be distinguished scientists and commentators who will tell us about the things we see, and will answer all our scientific questions. We will be exploring the depths of the oceans and the creatures who dwell there. We will be learning about the flora and fauna of different countries. We will be learning about the geology of the earth, and about astronomy and the wonders of the universe. We will be learning about the fundamental sciences of physics and chemistry, and about mathematics, which, to a great extent, is the language of the basic sciences. Of course, human beings not only learn about science, they also apply it. So we will learn about the world of manufactured objects and engineering. In fact, we will be made familiar with everything of the sciences which a non-scientist can be taught to appreciate. We will also be learning about medicine, which approaches the human body as an object to be learnt about in the same way that we learn about inanimate objects. We will derive great enjoyment from our visit to the world of science, and there are some observations which we shall make about it. During our visit, we were always observing things from the outside, or we were being told about things external to ourselves. Of course, a great deal of science is not to do with observing phenomena, but with explaining them. But this, too, can be regarded as learning about things external to ourselves. We can be detached, and it is right that we should maintain this detachment. We must realise that the detached consideration of phenomena external to us is of the very essence of the profession of science. Further, everybody was reasonably amicable, and any disagreements between people did not lead to hostility.

We will now visit our world where there are all manner of people. Any scientists we find are not there in a scientific capacity, but just as human beings. There are the great writers, philosophers, artists, musicians, and composers. There are religious leaders of all faiths, professional atheists, freethinkers, and politicians of every description. There are journalists, opinion-formers of all kinds, psychotherapists and psychoanalysts. There are tyrants, and the people they have oppressed, persecutors and those they have persecuted, gangsters, criminals and their victims. There are protagonists from every conflict there has ever been, loving couples and divided couples. And, above all, there are ordinary people, in far greater numbers than can possibly be counted.

Between all these people there will be every conceivable emotion possible: love and hatred, affection and indifference, emulation and envy, respect and disdain. People will feel love and affection towards some, but will feel animosity and hatred towards others. Our world is one where emotions flourish. Whereas there was a fair degree of harmony in the world of science, in our world there is the potential for conflict of the utmost ferocity and bloodshed.

Not only is our world a world of potential conflict, but it is also a world where the truth is manipulated by one set of people or another. It is never right to assume a respect for the truth in any section of humanity, but in the world of science, it is safer to assume it than elsewhere, provided that the science is not biased by human concerns. However, in our world respect for the truth can never be assumed, and that is one of its distinguishing characteristics. The reason for this is not mysterious. People have other desires than a respect for the truth, and sometimes these other desires override it partially or completely. People communicate with each other for a number of different reasons, and the assertion of the truth is just one of them.

Even when people try to assert the truth about something, there is a whole mass of ideas and considerations in the background influencing what they say. In the world of science, things can, to a large extent, be considered in isolation. In our world, the merits of a particular course of action or the truth of a particular statement tend to be considered in the context of a whole lot of other things which are psychologically connected to it, but not logically connected to it at all. People rarely consider a particular question on its merits, unconnected to how they think about other things. And that can be the case even with people who consider themselves unbiassed. Thus even when direct lies are avoided, the truth can be prevented from appearing.

Our world is a very political world. The national politics with its rival political parties, and the international world with its relations between the various countries, are only two of the spheres where what is essentially politics holds sway. There are few parts of our world where politics of one form or another does not make its presence felt. We are social beings, there are rivalries between us, and alliances. Our strivings for worldly success are deeply tinged with politics. Things are not isolated from one another in our world, to be managed without reference to anything else. That dispassionate outlook may be possible in science, but it is scarcely possible in our world.

We have a sophisticated world where concepts and ideas are abundant. The world of ideas expands our personalities. The world of science is also a world of ideas, and it has certainly expanded our horizons, but science is just one part of our enrichment by the world of ideas. We human beings are a reflective species, and we reflect on any number of things, including ourselves and our fellow creatures. We have intellects and we have emotions, and the two are very intertwined. That is why we sometimes have mental troubles.

In the world of science, we were observers and analysts. In our world, we are participants. We take part in a whole string of activities along with a lot of other people. And what we do is important to us as human beings, as are our relations with others. People may have experiences that lift us up, or experiences which put us down. We may go through the whole gamut of emotions, and there are reasons behind everything we do or say. Our behaviour may sometimes be bizarre, but it is never inexplicable. Here we are part of the action. People make decisions and do various things, many of which rebound upon us with consequences sought or unsought. We cannot say that anybody is mad in this world of ours, for there is a definite reason for every type of behaviour. We are rational beings, trying to react to any of life's vicissitudes in the way best suited to preserve our emotional equilibrium. Our reactions depend on what life presents us with. Of course, not everybody reacts the same to the same sort of stimuli. Life would be very boring if they did. Here, numerous lives come together, and interact with one another. The novelist, the journalist, the psychologist or psychotherapist, are welcome to enter our lives to record them or to help us, because they, too, are people, just the same as us.

9

Psychotherapy

Psychoanalysis And Psychotherapy

Psychoanalysis originated with Freud and his followers at the end of the 19th and the first half of the 20th century. It spread throughout the world, and particularly to the English-speaking countries. In some ways, it looks back to the moral treatment of the Tukes at the beginning of the 19th century. But unlike them, psychoanalysis possessed a substantial body of theory to back up its treatments. Today, orthodox psychoanalysis is not the only form of in-depth psychotherapy, but there is more similarity than difference between the different types of psychotherapy in practice. The great insight of Freud which permeates all of them is the existence of the unconscious, which influences people, though they may not be aware of it. We bury unacceptable thoughts and feelings in our unconscious, which a psychoanalyst or psychotherapist, acting as our friend, helps us to bring into the conscious mind. Another very important insight is that the communications and behaviour of those who come for therapy are taken absolutely seriously. Another insight is the fact that, for successful therapy, the therapist acts, to a certain extent, as a benign father or mother figure.

The advent of psychoanalysis and psychotherapy was perceived as a threat by a great many psychiatrists. This was especially the case with the advent of lay therapists. These persons were qualified in psychoanalysis or psychotherapy, but not in medicine. The success of these therapists implied that it was not necessary to be medically qualified to be a successful therapist. Many psychiatrists felt that they might be out of a job. They had justification for feeling this, for psychotherapy is popular,and it would be even more popular if it was made more financially affordable.

Thus, there arose a state of hostilities between the old psychiatry, which we will call biopsychiatry, which believed that mental illnesses were caused by abnormalities in the brain,and administered treatments such as drugs and ECT, and psychoanalysis and psychotherapy. The latter have been accused of not being relevant to extreme cases such as that of the psychotics, though in fact that is not true. The latter has also been accused of being very time-consuming, which puts off people who want a quick fix.

The threat of competition from psychotherapy has made the biopsychiatrists even more dogmatic and vociferous in their claims,and in their denigration of the former. In fact,all this is just propaganda churned out by biopsychiatrists wanting to preserve their jobs,and by the political and medical establishments and the drug companies.

The Reasonableness Of Psychotherapy

Psychotherapy is often referred to as the talking therapy. This is supposed to be disparaging. The assumption is that merely talking with someone could surely not cure anybody of anything. On reflection,you may think differently.

Talking with someone is a form of communication with them. It is perhaps the most important form of communication. Communication with other people has taken place continually since birth. It has increased in importance as the years have gone by. We would be very different beings without it. Without it,human beings would not be the same kind of creatures at all.

Of course,actions and experiences of a physical nature are

as important as communication with others. But it is by communication that we make sense of our experiences, and reflect upon them. If a counsellor or therapist is going to make a difference to how we view our experiences, it is by communicating with us that they are going to do it. The change in how we think about our experiences will be achieved, if at all, by a talking therapy.

Sessions with a psychotherapist will not be the first time that the persons receiving therapy have been influenced by what other people say to them. There will have been countless other communications with people throughout their lives. All of these will have affected them. The difference is that, with therapy, the clients have ideally a friend, who is not part of their lives, whose job it is to help them to get over their problems, and reach for something better.

There are types of talking therapy that aim to persuade people to change their behaviour in the present, rather than alter their perspective on their past. This can be behavioural therapy, which aims to change a person's behaviour by means of rewards and punishments, or it can be occupational therapy which aims to divert a person from their present emotional problems by giving them new occupations or amusements. Or the therapy may consist of giving practical advice to people about how to improve their lives. These therapies are valuable and have their rôles to play in the treatment of a client. But they are different from in-depth psychotherapy. They do not delve into the past so that the client can relive it, go beyond it, and grow into a more fulfilled person.

There is one type of occupational therapy which goes beyond being just an occupation to take the person's mind off his or her troubles. That is art therapy, where the person with troubles feels free to give expression to his or her traumas in disguised form in painting, sculpture, peotry, or music. Here, the art therapy is not just an enjoyable occupation, but is itself a form of in-depth psychotherapy. This art therapy has been used successfully with people suffering from combat stress from their experiences of war.

In-depth psychotherapy almost always takes a certain amount of time, and sometimes a considerable amount of time. It is not a quick fix. But the genuine relief of mental problems is never a quick fix, whatever method you employ, and it is an illusion to think it is. This is in contrast to many ailments in ordinary medicine, where a cure can often be effected reasonably quickly.

The lack of a quick fix for mental problems should come as no surprise. It has taken a number of years for the mental problems to come to the person's notice as problems. There will be the past events, and the person's reactions to them at the time. These reactions will be those that seemed best at the time. They were not the reactions that the person would make in his or her present state of mind. When the memories of all this surfaces to consciousness, it is not surprising that a certain amount of time is needed to resolve them. If strong emotions are involved, some time may pass between the intellectual remembering of a past event, and the complete remembering of it, along with its accompanying emotions.

Another problem with in-depth psychotherapy is that it is difficult to say precisely when a cure has been achieved. Much of the change brought about is a change in the inner life of the person, and this may not be obvious to a casual observer. Of course, if the mental problems of the person have been very severe, with a lot of adverse affect on behaviour, then a change will be apparent in the behaviour of the person after a comparatively short period of successful treatment. But, in any case, if the therapy has been beneficial, there will come a time when the client is sufficiently strong mentally to live his or her life without therapy. If both client and therapist are honest, they will realise this.

A person can derive help from a therapist, and that help can be very valuable, but the help should not swamp the person such that no true individual personality is allowed to emerge. Many artists go to an art college, but, if they are going to be any good, they need to wean themselves from the influence of the art college, and develop their own artistic personalities. The same applies to a person receiving therapy. Therapy is not a substitute for life, nor is it a valid alternative to it. Therapy is merely a help, though it may be a great help, and both therapist and client should think of it in those terms.

In-depth psychotherapy is part of the ordinary life of the individual concerned. Each individual has his or her own life, and value-judgements about it are for the individual alone to make. Cures such as are reported for physical ailments, and the scientific tests of cures associated with them, are not appropriate here. In-depth psychotherapy is to do with the subjective, rather than with the objective, which is preferred in the sphere of science. The success of a therapist will depend much more on the rapport which he or she manages to make with the client, and on the therapist's experience, rather than on the possession of an orthodox quasi-scientific body of knowledge.

10

Look Into Psychoanalysis

In the previous chapter, I have put forward the idea that seeking psychotherapy is a reasonable choice for a person suffering from mental problems. In this chapter, I shall take a look at psychoanalysis, and I shall deal with criticisms of it that people have sometimes made.

Though there was a dim awareness of the existence of the unconscious before Freud, it was Freud and psychoanalysis that first understood its supreme importance. Accordingly, events in the past history of a person, which are rejected by the conscious mind as being repugnant to it, remain in the unconscious until they can be induced to resurface into consciousness. Freud and many analysts used the interpretation of dreams and the technique of free association to bring this about. George Frankl and others also used a form of hypnosis.

But psychoanalysis not only posits the existence of the unconscious, but also puts forward the idea of the development of the sexuality of each person from infancy to adulthood, and stresses the supreme importance of this for the development of character. This acknowledgement of the sexual feelings of children was revolutionary in its time. If the feelings of the child are not acknowledged in the way they should be, the result can be mental problems including neurosis or psychosis. The origin of these may also be actual sexual or physical abuse of children, which happens all too frequently, and the way such abuse is responded to by parents and other adults. Traumas in adult life can also give rise to

47

mental problems, but usually the mind of an adult is that much stronger.

The rôle of the analyst in psychoanalysis is also very important. It is not sufficient that the things which have been repressed in the unconscious should be recalled and acknowledged intellectually. The emotions concerning these things need to be relived as well. For this, the support of the analyst is vital. George Frankl makes the point that it is no use for the analyst to be just an impassive observer. The analyst needs to be the client's friend, and to give emotional support.

There are a number of theoretical concepts in psychoanalysis. There are the oral stage, the anal stage, the early genital stage, the latency period, and the later genital stage at puberty in the sexual development of children. There is the Oedipus Complex and the Electra Complex. And there is the Ego, the Id, the Superego, and the Libido. All these concepts have a useful part to play in psychoanalysis. There is support for these concepts from the experiences of actual people. They are useful in describing the mental world of human beings. We have to realise that these concepts deal with fundamentals applicable to human beings in general. There may be some variations between different cultures. Nevertheless, these concepts make a far better attempt at describing the fundamentals of the human mentality than any other theories up to now, including psychiatry, which makes no serious attempt to do this at all.

To some critics, all this is not sufficiently scientific. But the same could be said about theoretical concepts in the social sciences, literature, or the arts. You cannot expect the scientific rigour of the physical sciences in the field of the mental and the subjective, whose existence is not really acknowledged by some scientific psychologists, anyway. The psychoanalytical concepts are helpful guidelines. With these guidelines in the background, it will be the experience of dealing with the problems of clients that will sharpen the skills of a psychoanalyst. Each client is unique, and every client will have a particular unique history. The psychoanalytical concepts are just helpful indications of what people may have in common.

Some people think that the rôle of the analyst means they impose a particular interpretation on the client. But the analyst need not tell the client what interpretation he or she is putting on the client's revelations from the unconscious. A good analyst will use discretion about this. Really, what is important is what the client thinks and feels, not what the analyst thinks. And a good analyst will acknowledge this.

To other critics, there is the fact that some psychoanalysts and psychotherapists have not behaved with professional integrity. But the same could said about every profession, without exception. That is why I do not pay much attention to the criticisms of Freud and psychoanalysis made by Jeffrey Masson. He was a university professor of Sanscrit who trained to become a psychoanalyst, and practised as such for a time. I feel, through reading his books, that he did not have any significant mental problems himself, and was therefore unable to empathise with those who had them. I feel that he was always an intellectual who looked at psychoanalysis from the outside, and that he did not really grasp what the whole enterprise was all about.

It is a very good thing if therapists have themselves had mental problems or some sort of difficulties in their lives, so that they can appreciate the mental distress of their clients and can empathise with them. The therapist will then understand why people wish to come for analysis. It is a requirement for a therapist to have a training analysis, so that he or she is aware of his or her own prejudices or hang-ups. The therapist also needs to know what happens in an analysis, what the procedure is.

The therapist may be the only person in the world to whom the client has confided certain things, and these things are confided to the therapist because he or she is outside the client's normal life, and because what is said will not be told to anybody else. In the course of therapy, a lot of things may emerge from the unconscious to be acknowledged by the conscious mind. This process may be painful, but it may also be liberating.

The relationship between therapist and client is of prime importance in psychoanalysis and psychotherapy. Obviously, if the therapy is going well, the therapist is bound to have some influence on the client. But provided the client is happy about this, then that is allright. There will probably have been many influences on the client in his or her life, such as family, friends, and colleagues at work. The influence of the therapist is just one of them. The success of the therapy may well depend on the client going to the right therapist, or at least avoiding going to one with whom he or she is not compatible. Also there are a number of different versions of psychotherapy, and the client needs to know what they desire from therapy.

Paddling Your Own Canoe

Psychotherapists are not the only people who have profound influence on the lives of individuals, and it is rather absurd to pretend that they are. The reason for their being resorted to is that the previous influences on the individual's life, though profound, were not beneficial, but damaging. Though an individual can be helped by a psychotherapist to bring to the surface of the mind things which have been repressed in the unconscious, the therapist also acts as a father figure or mother figure to the individual. It is, of course, the mother and father who, in every case where they are present, have a profound influence on the child, and through the child on the adult. The mutual influences of husband and wife on each other are also profound, unless the marriage is semi-detached and therefore, of lesser importance. What is at issue here is the prime importance of love.

We talk about a person's formative years, and that suggests that the person is being profoundly influenced by something, whether it be by other people or by experiences. The present mental state of a person at any particular time is the result of his or her reactions to the total life experiences up to that time. The reactions are those of a person with a certain inborn character reacting to the experiences, and the character of the person will change to a certain extent, and develop as their life proceeds.

The individual, in the course of his or her life, will have good experiences and bad experiences, and sometimes he or she may feel in an infinitely bad way. There may be somebody in their acquaintance who will come to the rescue, or this may not happen. If it does happen, the rescuer will be giving to the individual something of profound benefit. In these circumstances, a person who merely offered comfort of a trivial sort would be no use. A friend of mine had a very traumatic period in her life away from her family and in a strange land. The father of a friend of hers did come to the rescue, and pulled her through this very dark period of her life, so that she was able to move forward and get better. She was persuaded that life was still worth living, and was guided as to how to make the best of it. It is a bit of luck whether a rescue of this sort will occur. Sometimes it does, sometimes it doesn't.

In the case I mentioned just now, the rescuer was just an ordinary person with empathy, and not somebody qualified in psychotherapy. And in a great many situations in life, this will be the case. A great teacher may have profound influence. A bosom friend may be just what is required. Meeting the love of one's life may be a life-changing experience. There can be many such occurrences in a person's life. These must be contrasted with the many more encounters with other people, which can only be regarded as meaning little emotionally, and certainly not capable of rescuing the person from anything.

The need for recourse to a psychotherapist will arise, either when there is no rescuer of sufficient strength and commitment in sight, or when there is a real need to delve into the unconscious of a person, so that he or she can relive the traumas of the past and their emotional reactions to them, and go beyond them. It is the the perogative of the individual to decide whether this is the case, or not. If the decision is made to seek help, it is vital that they seek help from a psychotherapist, rather than from a psychiatrist with their physical and chemical remedies. And the would-be client should feel free to shop around in order to ensure that the pyschotherapist is compatible.

The individual personality is determined by the various decisions which he or she makes in his or her life. Some of these decisions may be good, and some bad. Nobody can get it right all the time. If too many of the person's decisions are made by other people, including therapists, then the development of an authentic individual personality is thwarted. Sooner or later, it must be acknowledged that this development is the object of the exercise. Further, the mental troubles of an individual should be acknowledged as part of what has made that individual have the personality which he or she has.

Psychotics

A lot of people have thought that in-depth psychotherapy was only suitable for neurotic clients of a fairly cultured milieu. In fact, people from all sections of the population, in addition to any practical problems which they may have, can also have severe psychological problems. It was also thought that psychotics were too disturbed to be treatable by psychotherapy. But, in fact, they can be so treated.

Bertram Karon and Gary Vandenboss have shown that it is certainly possible to give in-depth psychotherapy to psychotic patients. They were mainly dealing with schizophrenics. It is very rewarding to read their book *"Psychotherapy Of Schizophrenia"*. In every case, when they talked with the patients and thought about their symptoms in the light of the material that emerged in therapy, the pathological symptoms were always a natural result of their life histories, both in severity and in specific details. In all cases, the individuals had lived lives which we could not conceive of living without developing their symptoms. Every one of the symptoms of schizophrenia is meaningful, and is embodied in the life history of the patient.

What is apparent when giving therapy to psychotics is that the therapist must really want to help the client. The therapist needs to be extremely patient. A long time and many sessions may elapse before progress is made. Nevertheless, there will come a time when the client, though still disturbed, is no longer psychotic. Henceforth, the therapy will more closely resemble the therapy given to a non-psychotic client. To start with, the schizophrenic will be intensely frightened of everybody and everything. Such a client will need to be reassured that he or she is safe, and is not going to be killed. Also the behaviour of the psychotic will usually be more socially unacceptable than that of the average neurotic client, at least at the start. The therapist will need to be extremely tolerant. There is no doubt that giving psychotherapy to a psychotic is extremely demanding emotionally of the therapist. It is not surprising if the majority of therapists do not attempt it. But whereas they cannot be blamed if they admit that they do not want to do it, they can be blamed if they pretend that it is impossible, whereas, in reality, it is they themselves who are not capable of doing it.

In a study in America, schizophrenic clients who received even a small amount of psychoanalytical therapy (70 sessions over a 20 month period) showed less thought disorder (they were more able to think logically when they wanted to), spent much less time in hospital, and were able to live their lives more fully than those who had received medication. Further, these effects were not transitory, but became more marked, the longer the clients were followed up.

Another psychoanalyst who gave in-depth therapy to a few psychotics, and expressed interest in the possibility of more of this being done was George Frankl. He pointed out that the troubles of psychotics have their origins in a very early period of childhood, and that the characteristic of psychotics is the weak development of the ego. His treatment of them made extensive use of hypnosis.

I feel sure that there are in the world a sufficient number of people who, with appropriate training, would be willing and capable of giving in-depth psychotherapy to psychotics.

It must be stressed that psychotherapy never in itself does physical harm to the client. Sometimes, though rarely, a client may commit suicide and the therapist may be blamed for not having prevented it. But the suicide could well have happened anyway, and the client is a free agent. That is not the same as doing deliberate physical harm to the client. When we consider psychiatry, which is dominated by the medical model, we will find that physical harm is definitely done to patients. From the extreme case of lobotomy to ECT and to drug treatment, brain damage is part of the package, and in many cases, the brain damage is irreparable. That is never the case with psychotherapy of any kind, and that can never be emphasised enough. Criticisms of therapy can be met by therapists exercising integrity and common sense. Psychotherapy of one kind or another is the only external help that can be given to anyone in mental distress, which does no permanent harm, and which can bring inestimable benefit.

11

Alleged Dangers
Of The Mad

Those Who Are A Danger To Themselves

The justification which psychiatrists use for detaining people in institutions against their will is that they are a danger to themselves or others. In this section, I will discuss those who are just a danger to themselves. In short, I will be discussing suicide and attempted suicide.

In the past, there were religious sanctions against committing suicide. People who committed suicide were not allowed to be buried in consecrated ground. Usually today, that prohibition is waived by the fiction that they committed suicide while of unsound mind. But it is not hard to imagine circumstances where somebody might be perfectly rational and might wish to commit suicide. However, if you attempt to do so today, you are liable to be detained in a psychiatric institution against your will. This could be said to be infringing your human rights.

Further detaining someone and giving them drugs or ECT can as easily drive them to commit suicide as to prevent them doing so. Indeed, such action, with the purpose of saving them from death, actually diminishes their capacity to enjoy life.

If someone really wishes to commit suicide, they will find means of doing so. You cannot stop them. The ability to telephone the Samaritans organisation at any time of the day or night has probably stopped very many intended suicides from carrying out their intentions. In the long term, the wish to commit suicide can be changed, either by the action of life itself, or by successful psychotherapy. It would help if there were places of refuge to which emotionally fragile people could go without fear of being given ECT or drugs, but these are very rare at the present time. For this reason, the provision of such safe havens is a vital part of any good treatment of people with mental problems, and will be discussed at length later in this book. But every measure of help relies on the would-be suicide's cooperation.

Ultimately, you cannot stop someone committing suicide by the use of compulsion.

Those Who Are A Danger To Others

Nowadays, people charged with severe criminal offenses can plead that they were not responsible for their crimes by reason of being mentally ill. Whether they are or not is decided by a qualified psychiatrist. The plea of guilty but insane originated in the days when there was capital punishment for murder, and, if successful, resulted in saving the accused's life. Nowadays, if they are diagnosed as mentally ill, instead of going to prison, they go to a mental institution. That is supposed to be a preferable alternative. I don't think it is.

The important difference between persons imprisoned for their crimes, and persons confined to mental institutions for their alleged insanity, is that the former have definite rights, but the latter do not. Those in mental institutions are treated against their will, supposedly for their own good. They are entirely dependent on the inclinations of the psychiatrists. That is a very dangerous situation for anybody to be in. This is not the case with those in prison. There are objective legal criteria for how long a prisoner stays in prison. The length of stay of those in mental institutions depends on the decisions of the psychiatrists as to their mental conditions, which is far more subjective. The prisoner in prison is treated as a rational human being. He or she can even complain about his or her treatment. The psychiatric inmate is treated as irrational, therefore, their complaints are generally ignored.

There are other implications of the treating of violent criminals as insane. It couples together the two concepts of violence and insanity. It insinuates that those people confined in mental institutions are liable to be violent. In fact, the vast majority of mental patients are not violent.

But if we can no longer say that people accused of violent crimes are guilty but insane, what do we do with them? The answer is that we send them to prison, and treat them like other prisoners. But the cry will echo from the psychiatrists that we are not giving them any treatment. But the treatment given by the psychiatrists is not proper treatment. If treatment of any kind is to be given, then it should be requested by the person concerned. And psychotherapy should be available to any prisoner who requests it.

There is a further point, that until somebody has actually committed a criminal offence and been convicted of it, he or she cannot be imprisoned. If you suspect that someone may be about to commit an offence, then all you can do is watch the person, and perhaps see that they do not become employed by an institution where they come into contact with vulnerable people.

With respect to crime, the psychiatrists are not the only people who can decide to be lenient when it is fitting. Far from it! The judiciary is perfectly capable of leniency. In the case of violent crime, there can be mitigating circumstances, including self defence, provocation, accident, or even such a thing as a traumatic background. All these can be taken into consideration by a judge, and influence the sentence given.

If institutional psychiatry was no longer there, we would not be at the mercy of violent psychotics. If somebody is suspected of being violent, we keep him or her under suspicion. If somebody commits a violent crime or an offence giving grounds to think that they might be violent, then, if convicted, he or she is sent to prison. The whole point of sending somebody to prison is to protect the public. The length of sentence depends partly on the degree of danger the prisoner presents to the public when released. There is no reason why the absence of institutional psychiatry from the scene should increase the dangers to the public. In fact, the drug treatment that the psychiatrists are inclined to use could increase the violent tendencies of the prisoner, instead of abating them. And if we need advice about how violent a convicted criminal is likely to be, we could consult a criminologist just as well as a psychiatrist.

The rôle that psychiatrists have up to now played in the judicial system is not necessary. We can deal with violent offenders without it.

Mad And Bad

Some psychiatrists and members of the public think that being violent is itself a criterion of insanity.

Often people say, when they think of mass murderers or uniquely evil people such as Hitler, Stalin, or Pol Pot, that such people must be mad. The theory is that no sane man or woman would behave like they did. The concept of madness is brought in to distance ourselves from such people. The theory is that crimes against humanity, such as were tried at Nuremberg, were aberrations from the normal behaviour of human beings. Now it is true that crimes of a certain magnitude involving great numbers of victims do not happen everywhere, and they do not happen all the time. Nevertheless, there is a good deal of wishful thinking in the idea that these were completely irrational aberrations. The reasoning seems to be that it is natural for human beings to be benevolent, but unnatural for them to be cruel and violent. On the contrary we must realise that cruel and violent behaviour, though morally abhorrent, is not necessarily irrational, and is not necessarily uncommon.

The fact is that Hitler had a very flourishing career as dictator of Germany, and Mengele had a very flourishing career as a SS doctor and Nazi scientist. The same could be said of Stalin, Pot Pol, and thousands of others. The idea of killing these people is sensible. The idea of trying to change them by treating them as psychopaths is ludicrous. Their whole identities are bound up with what they did, including their crimes.

But supposing you had managed to approach these people before they had committed their crimes, would it not be appropriate to give them a bit of therapy? But I do not think that any of these people were disturbed in the sense that they had personal mental illnesses. And if they were psychologically disturbed, their disturbance was something which they had in common with a lot of other people who were involved in committing their crimes. What they did wrong was done in the company of a lot of other people who thought as they did, and the fault was in the fundamental ideals motivating them. Of course, we can ask what was the psychology behind the ideals motivating these people. That is an interesting investigation which has been undertaken by distinguished psychoanalysts, and I will say more about it later in this section, but it does not alter the fundamental point I am making in this paragraph.

It is interesting that psychiatry has often been used as a weapon by the oppressors against the oppressed, but never, as far as I know, by the oppressed against their oppressors.

The correct way of regarding mental illnesses or mental problems is that they are debilitating conditions. To understand how a mental illness can be described as a debilitating condition, I would say that it is metaphorically similar to how a person would feel if he or she had got a stretch of rope, and tied themselves in knots. In this situation, whatever you want to do in life or whatever kind of life you want to lead, you are in some degree restricted. You are not really the person you want to be. That is why you would want help from a therapist, and why it makes sense for you to have therapy. If you are leading a successful life of crime, your choice to do so may be reprehensible, but you are not handicapped in living such a life. If you were handicapped by a so-called mental illness, you would not be able to lead such a successful life of crime.

Some people find it difficult to believe that certain people may choose a life of crime. Crime can bring rich rewards, as it does to Mafia bosses. These people have chosen their way of life voluntarily. The acceptability of violence may be part of the character of certain people. The case of paedophiles has been much in the news lately. But just as certain people choose to go in for large scale burglary for the sake of the money involved, so another set of people go in for paedophile type crimes for the gratification involved. Totalitarian dictators act the way they do because of their love of power. In doing so, these types are totally disregarding the well-being of their victims. But the paedophile or the sex murderer, the burglar, and the totalitarian dictator, have chosen to act in the way they do. They could have chosen to act otherwise. In reality, people are deterred from committing violent crimes by the high probability of being caught, convicted, and punished.

There are an enormous number of different people in the world. Some of these people we will respect and admire, others we will disapprove of. Some of the latter will be criminals in a moral sense, even if they have not actually been convicted of anything by the laws of the land.

But someone will say that in their innermost beings, everybody would prefer to love their fellow human beings, and behave accordingly. I think that that is true. But, as I said earlier, the investigation into the deeper motivations of successful perpetrators of crime has been undertaken by psychoanalysts. In this regard, the psychological sickness of various societies have to be considered as well as the psychological sickness of individuals. George Frankl has dealt with these questions in his books. The understanding of these deeper motivations will take a long time to penetrate into the culture, and influence it. In many ways, such an enterprise is similar to the idealistic commitment to persuade people to be virtuous. This is an idealist dream. We may work towards bringing this situation about, but it is certainly not the case now. We may feel a commitment to persuade people to be virtuous, but this will only ever have partial success. The fact that not everybody will be persuaded to be virtuous is part of the human condition. Meanwhile, the different lives which people lead are the product of their free choice.

We have to accept that it is right and proper to judge people. To think, as B.F. Skinner does in "*Beyond Freedom And Dignity*", that we can avoid doing this by renaming the actions of people as sane or insane, to be determined by psychiatrists, is a dereliction of our duties as human beings. This goes against the entire concept of free will, and threatens us with the medicalization of our entire society. This is extremely dangerous, and must be seen for the danger it is, since the medicalization of our society means a new tyranny. We are not so fond today of the old moral concepts of good and evil, merciful and cruel, true and false, and right and wrong. But we cannot do without them. If we try to do so, we submit to the tyranny of the experts, who, whatever people may think, are not infallible. Unfortunately, the experts may think they are, and, if we are not careful, they may be supported by the law of the land. And that makes them more formidable opponents than the old moral censors. We must at all times uphold the concept of individuals having free will. Sometimes we may have cause to punish them severely for some of the choices they make, but we should respect the fact that they have a free choice. In doing so, we respect them as individuals.

This wish to replace our old ways of looking at things in terms of morality by a new pseudo-scientific ordering of everything is part of a particular modern illusion. Some years ago, after the end of the Cold War, an American academic stated that it marked the end of history. He has surely been proved wrong. Contrary to what some people believe, there have always been struggles between people, usually accompanied by violence, and probably there always will be. Certainly, there will always be problems. No sooner is one problem overcome, but another problem arises to take its place. The matron of a London hospital told my mother that cancer might be overcome, but some other disease would arise to take its place. It is characteristic of problems that they are not predicted before they confront us. That exposes the futility of trying to make our lives fullproof against adversity by pseudo-scientific controls. We would do best to admit our limitations, and accept human free will.

12

Psychiatric Patients

The relatives of psychiatric patients

The relatives of psychiatric patients are not necessarily good friends to them. In America, the National Alliance For The Mentally Ill (NAMI), which is an organisation composed of the parents and other close relatives of psychiatric patients, is supportive of all the treatments such as drugs and ECT, and even, on occasion, lobotomy, which the psychiatrists give their patients. It is totally in league with the biopsychiatrists. Some people will even go so far as to use biopsychiatry as a weapon against family members whom they dislike or wish to push aside. A really horrific case of a relative using psychiatry for coercion is reported by Thomas Szasz in his book *"Coercion As Cure"*. A 12-year-old child called Howard Dully was given a lobotomy by the American lobotomist Walter Freeman after his stepmother complained that he was defiant. Howard's mother had died of cancer when he was five. His father remarried, and his stepmother hated him, and would do anything to get rid of him. She pressured his father to agree to the operation. By some miracle, the operation did not turn him into a zombie, but he said, "Ever since my lobotomy, I've felt like a freak, ashamed. I'll never know what I lost in those ten minutes with Dr Freeman and his ice pick". Fortunately, that is an extreme case, but it just shows what a lethal weapon biopsychiatry can be when it is used by unscrupulous relatives. Lucy Johnstone, in her book *"Users And Abusers Of Psychiatry"*, describes examples of women, who are exhausted and fed up with being the universal workhorse for their families, being placed in the psychiatric system, where the psychiatrists have no sympathy for their predicaments, but just give them drugs or ECT, and entirely side with the families.

NAMI is not so keen on psychotherapy. The reason is this. If people with mental problems receive psychotherapy, a lot of memories may come to the surface which are derogatory of the parents or spouses or other close relatives. The latter do not like this. And if they are sufficiently ruthless, they will do everything possible to prevent this occurring. They would like to preserve the image of themselves as supremely virtuous, and to maintain the person with mental problems in whatever rôle in which they present no threat. As a matter of fact, though some things may have been the fault of close relatives, some things may have been due to adverse circumstances or outsiders, where none of the relatives can be blamed. However, the biopsychiatrists, who have practically taken over the profession in America, do not go in for psychotherapy, and give their patients drugs or ECT, which tend to sweep all these traumatic memories under the carpet.

People tend to have certain rôles in life, and the family or even the workplace revolves around each person behaving in the way in which he or she is expected to behave. If a person has mental troubles or a mental breakdown, this system is disrupted, and the others, unless they are tolerant types or have great psychological awareness, do not like it. Some of the other members of the family may regard the situation in the same way as when the car breaks down. When that happens they send it to a garage which diagnoses the fault, repairs it, and returns it to its owner in a comparatively short time. These people may want a quick fix for the family member with mental troubles, in the same way as they would want a quick fix for the car with mechanical troubles. They are content if the psychiatrist takes the person with mental troubles, gives him or her drugs or ECT, and returns him or her to them to fulfil the same rôle as before. These people are not keen on the person having a long period of therapy, with the possible result that they are no longer content to play their rôle in the way they did in the past. Moreover, if anger against family members should arise in the course of the therapy, they will like this even less.

The family members described above are being ruthless. Certainly, they should not use psychiatry as a weapon against their relatives. Ideally, they should be in favour of the person with problems having therapy, and should be prepared to adapt themselves to the new emerging personality that comes into being after a period of time. Or when it is the family circumstances that are responsible for one person being designated as ill, they should ideally be prepared to change things for that person's benefit. However, far too many people are not willing to do this, and they collude with the biopsychiatrists to prevent it.

These family members are very much to blame, but they would have no power to act in the way that they do if they were not supported by institutional psychiatry. Biopsychiatry is being used in the quarrels of everyday life to coerce vulnerable people.

Sometimes when a married couple are living together, and the children have left the nest, one of them may get seriously depressed. This will not only be a great misfortune for the sufferer from depression, but will also put a great strain on the other one, who will have to put up with someone suffering from depression. If a psychiatrist has been called in, the carer may very well collude in whatever treatment he or she prescribes, even though such treatment may be very harmful to the sufferer in the long term. There again, the really harmful element in the situation is the biopsychiatrist. If psychotherapy was involved, there would be no danger of the sufferer from depression actually being harmed.

One good way of dealing with the families of people with mental troubles is to give social therapy to the family, as well as to the person with the troubles. This approach has been carried out a number of times, and has improved family situations greatly. Often the family set-up is the cause of the trouble, with one person singled out as being more mentally sick than the others. But they all have problems. In such a case, giving social therapy to the family as a whole is often very productive.

The parents of psychiatric patients often themselves have mental problems which were responsible for them behaving the way they did to their children. So the hostile attitudes towards their children receiving psychotherapy may be due to the fact that they are unwilling to confront their own mental problems. In fact, there is a hereditary factor here, but not in the way people generally think of heredity. It is not a matter of inherited genes, but of parents passing down to their children the upbringing which they had themselves. This factor in the situation should always be borne in mind. The only solution is to continually campaign to make people aware of psychological problems, not for the purpose of dealing with them by drugs, but for the purpose of understanding them properly.

The Predicament Of Psychiatric Patients

If people have been damaged physically by an assailant, their attitudes will be relatively straightforward. They will not shrink from proclaiming their injuries to the world, and demanding redress. But for patients who have been damaged by psychiatric treatments, it is not so simple. They will often try and deny the fact of the damage, even though it may be obvious to old friends. The attitude is understandable. Acknowledgement would be too painful.

People who are confined to mental institutions against their will as psychiatric patients have two factors against them. They start off in a vulnerable emotional state before they enter the institution, and the psychiatric treatments and their general feelings of powerlessness in the institution make this worse. They may not be inclined to make complaints, even if they were listened to. They may just resign themselves to conforming, for fear of being victimised if they complain. In addition, these patients may be comparatively ignorant, both of the dangers confronting them, and of anything they can do to better the situation.

Fortunately, there are very brave and strong individuals who, after they have been released from mental institutions, decide to fight against the psychiatric treatments that have damaged them, and to help others who have experienced the same. Hence we have the Survivors movements. Such movements have given quite a lot of support to their fellow survivors and to anybody in danger of getting into the hands of the psychiatric establishment. Among other things, they have established safe havens for vulnerable people to come and stay.

But some people who have been psychiatric patients and have experienced bad treatment will just lie low and pretend that the whole thing never happened. The only thing that could really change this would be the end of the present condition of the psychiatric establishment.

There is another misfortune suffered by psychiatric patients in addition to any debilitating treatment they may have received, and that is the acquisition of a psychiatric record. However, much of a recovery a person makes from their period of mental distress, the fact of their having been had a psychiatric classification will always remain on their medical record, and will count against them in such matters as job applications. Thus the institution of official psychiatry serves to stigmatise people.

Apart from the ex-patients who have suffered from official psychiatry, there are some people who have actually done everything possible to ensure that they will be admitted as psychiatric patients. This sounds bizarre. But a psychiatric hospital does look after you in every way. It relieves you of the need to make decisions for yourself. It also provides a certain amount of company. To some people, this can be preferable to the life which they could expect to live in the outside world, and the obedient taking of medication can be a price which they are willing to pay. This is a totally unadventurous choice, since they will not expand themselves in any way by taking it. However, that is what some people do. Lucy Johnstone describes people who do this in her book. In any new system of mental health care that we could envisage, the giving of practical help in improving the lives of these people would be a necessary part.

13

Science

Today, we live in a scientific age. Previous periods of human history were dominated by hereditary rulers and by religions of various kinds. The claims to legitimacy of both have been strongly disputed in the last few centuries, and neither of them, at least in the West, possesses the power they once had. Science has, in many ways, stepped into the breach. The popular attitudes towards it are quite interesting.

Many people are thrilled by science, and some are bored by it. Most people are reluctant to make their own investigations as to what the scientific position on any particular topic actually is, but accept blindly what the scientific experts are assumed to say. The veneration for authority, which previously was given to religious leaders or to hereditary rulers, is now given to scientists, regardless of what they say or recommend. The fact that science, at its best, can only tell you what is the case, and not what you should do about it, is ignored. If some scientists are to blame for this situation, the public is even more to blame.

The deference to scientific experts is given because of some official accreditation which they possess. The average member of the public has not either the will or the ability to go beyond the credentials and to examine the intricacies of the point in question. The fact that some official body has given their recognition to an expert counts for everything.

The history of science is thought of mainly as a history of successes. The failures, the false theories, and the red herrings that crop up from time to time are forgotten and ignored. This does not matter much in branches of science remote from human concerns, but when the issues to be considered lie in areas not so remote, it can matter considerably.

The pure activity of the scientist searching for the truth and only the truth, and not embellishing it or going beyond it, commands our wholehearted veneration. But science and scientists have been with us for quite some time now, and they have become very much part of our world. And just as religion, though purporting to concern itself with eternal verities, became corrupted by the ways of the world, so some scientists, in their turn, have become corrupted. Not everything that springs from the utterings of our scientific experts is uninfluenced by human partiality, political biases, or economic self-interest.

The history of medicine, in particular, consists of failures as well as successes. It is distinguished by the combination of the insatiable desire of patients for a relief from their sufferings, and the frequent inability of the doctors at any particular time to provide it. Unfortunately, patients are generally unwilling to be satisfied with an honest confession of inability to help.

It is the contention of this book that psychiatry is bogus as a profession and as a branch of medicine. But it is not alone in this respect. There was phrenology, which was bogus, but did not do much harm. And, to strike a more serious note, there was eugenics. Under the influence of eugenics, a large number of people designated as mentally ill or defective were killed in Nazi Germany. This goes to show that large numbers of highly qualified people can get things drastically wrong.

Psychiatry came into being as fulfiling the dual function of jailer and doctor. And the studies of the affects of this or that remedy which it has commissioned are highly suspect. Indeed, psychiatry shows that you can ape the trappings of science while disregarding the essentials.

Firstly, there is no objective test as to whether anybody has any of the conditions categorised as mental illnesses. The only evidence for a particular condition is the person's behaviour. This is not the case in ordinary medicine.

Secondly, there is no objective test as to whether anybody has been cured of any of these mental conditions. This, again, is not the case in ordinary medicine. Psychiatric treatments such as drugs or ECT can be pretty debilitating. As well as dampening the entire personality, they will dampen the symptoms considered as indicative of mental illness. The patient will be less emotional about it. Possibly that factor, together with a partial return to normal life, will constitute a cure in the eyes of the psychiatrists. What is not asked, and this is the really important question, is what the patient felt about it. The inner life of the person, which is really what a mental illness is all about, is ignored. And, the long-term future of the patient, which may be damaged by the drastic psychiatric treatments, is ignored too.

Often it is claimed in the psychiatric literature that one or other of the designated mental illnesses are genetic in origin. This is supposed to bring great joy to the biopsychiatric camp. But since no mental illness has been proved to have a biological origin, and since the psychiatric diagnoses for mental illnesses are vague and subjective, it is very difficult to see what exactly is being passed from one generation to another by genetic means. It may be the case that some inclination to have mental problems may be passed on genetically. But this may just amount to an inclination to have greater sensitivity than normal. Such an inclination would only favour the development of mental problems if the life circumstances of the person pushed the person in that direction. Therefore, no notice need be taken of claims for the genetic origin of mental illness. These claims are either false, or else they are claims of something so general as to be almost worthless.

If mental illness does not lie within the field of medicine, that is a reversal of the way things seemed to be going for quite some time. The phrase, the inexorable progress of science, comes to mind. The idea was that the success of the exact sciences in the fields of the physical, chemical, and biological would, in time, also stretch to things mental. Some people saw no reason why it should not. They could see no snags. But there are snags. Even in physics there is the Heisenberg uncertainty principle, according to which you cannot determine both the position and the velocity of an atomic particle at the same time. In regard to things mental, this uncertainty is magnified many times over. Basically, you cannot eliminate bias when one human being is considering the affairs of another, and you cannot predict in detail how the life of another person, left to their own free will, is going to unfold in the future. When you come up against the human personality, the exact sciences have come up against the buffers.

It is true that behind all our mental activities are the workings of our brains. But the dualism between the physical and the mental is different from the way it was sometimes thought of in the past. Using computer terminology, the brain of a person is the hardware. The thoughts, memories and feelings of the person are the software. Mental problems and mental illnesses relate to the software. Physical illnesses of the brain, and brain damage, relate to the hardware. The biopsychiatrists try to treat problems of the software by fiddling about with the hardware. The only result has been not to cure anything, but to destroy it.

If the pretensions of psychiatry are bogus, what is the case with psychotherapy. Helping somebody to unravel his or her mental problems and mental distress bears a strong analogy to detective work, as depicted in detective stories. With some writers of this genre there is a strong psychological element. But what is implied in the thrilling detective story is the delving beneath appearances to find out who the real culprit was. In good psychotherapy of someone in mental distress, there is the delving beneath appearances to reveal hidden episodes of the past, and the facilitating of the emergence of a new confident person at the end of the story. If anything in this field can be said to exude the true spirit of science, then it is psychotherapy.

14

The Mind

People often pay little attention to what is going on in the mind of others; what they are thinking and feeling can remain a closed book to them. They will associate with them, either in the workplace, or in their leisure. But their association can be on the surface, either for playing games or other activities together, or indulging in social pleasantries. Such association will tell each of them a bit about the other person, but it will generally not tell them a great deal.

People have personalities, life histories, accomplishments which they are proud to possess, and emotions of joy and sorrow. Above all, they have memories, so that their present is connected to their past, and they have ambitions for the future. All these things mean a great deal to them, so that to be deprived of any of them would be like the experience of loss on the amputation of a limb, and could perhaps be a more severe loss than the latter.

However, although all these things mean a great deal to the person to whom they belong, they may mean very little to casual acquaintances, and surprisingly little, even to close friends or relations. To other people, what matters about a person is how he or she relates to them, how he or she performs in the struggles of life, and their success or failure in fulfiling the rôle into which life has cast them. To the outside world, a person's behaviour is what is important.

People are judged by their behaviour in the various contexts in which their lives revolve. They are judged by how they interact with their colleagues in the workplace, and by how they perform the various tasks set before them. At home, they are assessed on how they perform in the rôles of sons or daughters, husbands or wives, or fathers or mothers. In each case, it is how others perceive them that is registered in how the public regard them. What the individuals themselves feel about their lives and things in general is something that most people do not bother to ask, unless they happen to have the desire and the ability to sense beneath the surface veneer which the individuals present to the world.

To a certain type of scientifically-minded observer, a person's inner life or mind is most inconvenient. It is vague, nebulous, unexpected, and disorderly. The trouble with a person's mind is that you cannot put your finger on it. It does not fit easily into the kind of categories in which items in the other sciences are accustomed to be put. There are some people, including academics, who do not appear to believe in the inner life of the mind. Among them in different ways are Gilbert Ryle in his book, "*The Concept Of Mind*", and Susan Blackmore in "*The Meme Machine*". Such people, while trying to be clever, are totally ignorant of the concerns which I have expressed in this book. If you have no mental troubles and are not in danger of falling into the hands of biopsychiatry, you need not pay much attention to the mind. But if you are not in that fortunate position, the mind will be very important to you indeed.

Of course, some people have attempted to describe the real personalities and the real minds which individuals possess. Such are the great writers and journalists. Psychotherapists and gurus of various kinds have also attempted to do this. And they have done this sort of thing with a fair amount of success. Ordinary people, too, have from time to time shown talent in understanding the minds and personalities of others. But in so far as any of this is recorded in writing, it is not presented in the scientific format familiar to academics.

In my opinion, psychiatrists probably have a very mundane view of people and their minds. They would recognise a genius, since by the time he or she is acclaimed as a genius, the acclamation is general, and they would not wish to be out of step with the majority. But the idea that each individual is a complicated creature, and in some ways has the mark of genius in them, is to most psychiatrists, an alien concept. They emphasise acceptable behaviour and the fulfilment of social functions, and they do not concern themselves with the inner mind of a person. But it is the inner mind which gives birth to all the individuality and uniqueness of a person, though the outward expression of this is in behaviour. And it is the inner mind which is at risk of being damaged by the treatments of the biopsychiatrists. The inner mind is acknowledged by in-depth psychotherapy, but biopsychiatrists are no good at that.

A number of people come into the public eye on account of accomplishments of one kind or another. They have shown considerable merit in particular fields of activity. They have reached these heights of success after a long period of preparation. These people deserve credit for their success obtained through hard work in getting as far as they have, but the types of mind and the variety of ideas which they possess are shared by a much larger group of people who do not put in the hard work that they do and, therefore, do not have their success. Carrying this thought to its logical conclusion, we can say that in every human being there is something unique, and in every human being, there is the spark of genius. But if you persist in regarding a person as no more than how he or she appears at a particular time, you will be blind to this. A person is a combination of three things: a past, a present, and a future. He or she has memories, present experiences, and aspirations for the future, about which another human being has only very limited knowledge. A spectator, viewing a person just as he or she appears at the present time, may be blind to that person's past, and also to that person's future.

15

Brain Damage

In the previous chapter, I have reflected on the mind and how it does not command the respect it deserves, not only from psychiatrists, but also from people at large. This has had grave consequences. Coupled with the demarcation of those designated as mad as totally different from the rest of us, it has allowed biopsychiatrists to inflict brain damage on these helpless people.

If a person has severe brain damage, particularly if the person is prevented by the brain damage from acting reasonably normally in social situations, then people who meet the person will notice this, and will probably be rather shocked. But when the brain damage does not prevent the person from acting superficially as normal, then people will not notice anything wrong. The fact that the person may have lost treasured memories or particular skills which they once possessed will not make an impact on outsiders. If they are told about it, they may express sympathy. If, on the other hand, a person has sustained a severe physical injury, such as loss of a limb or loss of sight or hearing, then the consciousness of the person's injury will make an immediate impression. Injuries to the brain do not leave a visible mark. Therefore, they can be inflicted more easily. This is reflected in the willingness of psychiatrists to prescribe drugs which act as chemical straight-jackets, whereas they refrain from putting psychiatric inmates in actual straight jackets, which they would have done in the past. The fact that actual straight-jackets do far less harm than chemical ones is disregarded, because the latter are less visible and so less disturbing to onlookers. Another aspect of brain damage is that most people who have experienced it, especially if it has been caused by psychiatric treatment, will attempt to deny it, since to acknowledge such an irreparable loss would be too painful.

We can assemble any gathering of people. Let them be writers, artists, musicians, scientists, academics, judges, politicians, financial wizards, and administrators. Let them be athletes, footballers, ballet dancers, television personalities, actors, or just plain ordinary people. In the case of all of them, whatever other part of their bodies they use in their lives, the most important organ of all for all of them is the brain.

If somebody has actual damage to the brain, or a genuine brain disease, then it is necessary to do everything possible to repair the damage, or alleviate it in some way. This is the job of a neurologist. But to inflict brain damage on a brain which is physically undamaged is an outrage. It is an affront to all of us. It shows total disregard of all the achievements of the human race in every sphere, because all these achievements are the work of brains. It shows total disregard and lack of respect for the thoughts and feelings which comprise the inner lives of every single one of us.

Today, we pride ourselves on not tolerating wrongs and abuses which we would have tolerated in the past. If, then, there is any spirit of integrity left in us, we should make it clear that the infliction of brain damage for any reason is completely unacceptable. The pretence that such an action could actually do anybody any good is complete humbug, and should be dismissed by all civilised people as a most atrocious lie.

16

Desirable Objectives

The Patient's Friend

There is the ideal of the good doctor as the patient's friend. It is a noble ideal. It combines with the Hippocratic Oath to define the proper medical ethics binding on the profession.

A person's solicitor or the barrister defending him or her in a court of law is in a similar position. While neither of them would sanction a client deliberately committing a crime in front of them, in every other respect, and especially with regard to confidentiality, each of them is the patient's friend.

For members of the Roman Catholic Church, their father confessor is in a similar position. In that case, the point about confidentiality is even stronger. In no circumstances can a father confessor relate what has been told to him in the confessional.

In the case of a doctor, the ideal of him or her being the patient's friend has become a bit blurred nowadays. In practice, it may depend on the amount of time he or she can give the patient, which in the case of the National Health Service (NHS) may be limited, as also on the conscientiousness of the particular doctor. Moreover, today, medicine has become increasingly technical, which may give both patient and doctor the feeling that a rapport between them is less important. Nevertheless, if a doctor actually harmed the patient, this would be looked upon as an unfriendly act.

For those who work for the NHS, they have a dual rôle of being the friends of the patients, and also employees of the state. Morally, they should be principally the friends of the patients. Nevertheless, since they are paid by the state and not by the patients, this dual rôle could bring problems. However, compared with psychotherapy, the problems this could give rise to in medicine need not be too many or too serious.

Psychotherapists of all descriptions, including psychiatrists who practice as psychotherapists, are ideally supposed to be the patient's friend. For therapists, the confidentiality required is virtually the same as that of a father confessor hearing a confession in the Roman Catholic Church.

It is absolutely essential that psychotherapists should be their clients' friends. They should not be employees of the state, and they should not be paid by the state, either. We may ask how the bills for this are going to be paid if the client is poor or out of work. People who have mental problems should be enabled by financial help from the state to pay for sessions with a psychotherapist of their choice if they so choose. But it should be entirely their decision as to whether they go to a psychotherapist, and, if so, which one they go to. In this way, we can ensure that psychotherapists are first and last the friends of their clients, which it is essential that they should be.

But why is it so essential that a psychotherapist should be the client's friend? It is because, apart from any expertise or experience, it is the prime job of the therapist to be such a person. The therapist may be the one person in the world to whom the client can disclose his or her most intimate secrets. They are friend of the friendless and the helper of the helpless, the one person in the client's life who does not have an axe to grind in the context of that life. The therapist's loyalty to the client must supercede all other loyalties except for the personal loyalties of the therapist's own life. It necessitates that they must not be paid by the state, or by anyone else but the client.

Availability Of Psychotherapy

Psychotherapy should be available for all those who wish to embark upon it. In the television program, "The Apprentice", in 2011 one of the candidates had a degree in Entrepreneurship. This did not go down very well with Lord Sugar, who is a top entrepreneur, but has no degrees. This shows the longing of people to have an official qualification for something, however inappropriate it is for the thing in question. There remains the question whether it is important to have a recognised qualification for giving psychotherapy. The answer is that the qualification itself is not important, but is merely a convenience. But it is important that the therapist should have studied the subject, and is not just a benevolent good listener, though such a person would be better than somebody who does harm to the client, such as a biopsychiatrist.

The essentials for a person to be capable of giving good psychotherapy are these:-

1) The client must make the decision to embark on therapy entirely voluntarily.

2) Therapists should have had psychotherapy themselves, and if the therapist is going to give in-depth psychotherapy, then he or she should have had in-depth psychotherapy themselves.

3) He or she should always remember that they are first and last the patient's friend. Whatever other allegiance the would-be therapist has to any organisation, political or religious, for example, must be put aside for the duration of therapy sessions. Likewise, the therapist should be the friend of the patient rather than the patient's relatives.

4) The therapist must possess the ability to see more in the client than the particular persona which the client presents to the therapist at the start of therapy. The whole point of therapy is to enlarge the life possibilities of the client, as well as helping the client through the sticky patch in his or her life at the moment.

5) The therapist should have a natural interest in people, and a curiosity about them, and a natural talent for dealing with them.

6) The therapist should have studied the subject in depth. But more important than anything is that the therapist should have a skill and aptitude for therapy. As I have said elsewhere, it would help if the therapist had had difficulties, or even traumas, in their life before commencing this work. That would enable the therapist to understand the situation of the client.

People with these prerequisites for giving psychotherapy may be found among all sections of the population. You do not have to come from a particularly well-educated social milieu to give good psychotherapy. People from any section of the population should be able to go to a psychotherapist of their choice if they so desire, and receive therapy at a cost that they can afford.

Therefore, the possession of a qualification in psychotherapy is only a guide for the prospective client. The real test comes with the client's experience of the therapy. Does the client regard the therapist as someone he or she can regard as a friend? Does the client feel that he or she is deriving benefit from the therapy sessions? If the client feels that they are not deriving benefit from a particular psychotherapist, then it may be best for the client to try someone else.

Safe Havens

Numerous people who experience severe mental distress want a place of refuge from their ordinary lives, but do not want to put themselves in the hands of the psychiatric profession, or go to mental hospitals which they have every reason to distrust and fear. The best option would be for them to go to a safe haven, if one exists, to which they can gain access. Hence there is a need for safe havens.

Residential safe havens should be run either by people who have had experience of mental distress themselves, or by ordinary people with a great deal of sympathy and tolerance. Under no circumstances should they be psychiatrists or employees of the mental health establishment. If once such people are allowed into the running of the safe haven, then it would become a mental hospital in all but name, run by the mental health professionals. However, the carers should not administer treatment themselves, least of all drug treatment. Treatment should be carried out by therapists visiting the safe havens if necessary, or more normally by the clients going to therapists for treatment. In all cases, treatment would have to be desired by the client. The atmosphere of the safe havens needs to be democratic, informal, and congenial, with no distinction between those in mental distress and the carers. The ideal safe haven is well described in a chapter entitled "The Duty Of Community Care: The Wokingham MIND Crisis House" by Pamela Jenkinson in the book "This Is Madness" edited by Craig Newnes, Guy Holmes and Cailzie Dunn.

Sometimes, the safe haven functions as a pleasant place to go to, where they are received by sympathetic people, and where they can pass the time resting, reading, talking to other people in the same predicament, and perhaps playing cards or billiards. They could actually sleep in a bed-and-breakfast place associated with the safe haven. Many people, even when they are in a condition of acute mental distress, can look after themselves, and can make their own decisions. For such people, the job of the safe haven is essentially to give moral support and empathy, and to give them the opportunity, if they so wish, to meet people in the same sort of condition as themselves.

Should anybody ever be referred to one of these safe havens compulsorily? This is a difficult question. Some people at some time in their lives can be in a psychotic state, and it could be in their best interest to go to a safe haven, whether they particularly wanted to or not, to avert immediate catastrophe.

But if they absolutely refused to go to a safe haven, I think that their wishes should be respected.

Appropriate work or occupational therapy should be available for the inmates to do while they are at the safe haven. If they can earn money for any work which they do, this might be beneficial for their development and for the success of any therapy they are receiving. It might give them a feeling of independence.

It is very important that these safe havens bear no resemblance to the mental hospitals that we are familiar with. The safe havens should be places entirely for the benefit of the inmates, who go to them as a refuge from their ordinary lives. From what I have said about the people who would be in charge of the safe havens and about the voluntary nature of any treatment, the difference should be clear.

To safeguard the safe havens as places totally different from the mental hospitals, their funding as I have already said, should be principally from voluntary contributions. They should not be financed by the state, though they should enjoy the status of registered charities, and possibly the purchase of their actual premises could be helped by donations from the local authorities. There should be no possibility of the state interfering with either the running of them, or with their existence.

Practical Therapy

There are a lot of people whose essential problem is that they have been overwhelmed by the difficulties and tribulations of their present lives. They may not need or desire to have psychotherapy, but they do want help with their practical problems. There has been some effort to deal with such people, but it needs to be increased. Really, the first thought to spring to mind when somebody has mental troubles should be whether their present life situation is the principal cause of the trouble. The interaction of adverse life situations and mental troubles has been well described by Lucy Johnstone in her book.

It is essential that the persons giving such help should be, first and last, the friends of the client, and not just employees of the psychiatric establishment. If they are the latter, there is always the risk that they might at some stage use the authority of the psychiatric establishment against the client. So, just as in the case of the psychotherapist, the social worker helping the client with practical problems must be the client's friend. Also, just as any good psychotherapy has to be desired by the client, so the client should be totally free to reject any advice given or course of action suggested by the social worker. The present position, where the social worker is under the authority of the psychiatrist, is unnecessary and detrimental to the interest of the client.

The skills needed for such a social worker are knowledge of the sort of problems facing the client and the capability to deal with them, as well as general friendliness, tolerance, and ability to deal with people. A formal qualification in social work should be advisable, but not essential. An older person with experience of life could be a good candidate for it. Social work like psychotherapy is a personal skill which some people have, rather than the possession of a body of knowledge.

Alongside social workers to help people with their practical problems, there needs to be the back-up support of public money for housing and other amenities.

17

The Future Of Psychiatry

The Politics Of Psychiatry

The behaviour of the psychiatric profession and of most psychiatrists from the earliest times to the present day has been political. Claims to benefit the patient and claims to be scientific are best thought of as adjuncts to essentially political behaviour. And if you ask what the motivation behind this political behaviour was, it was the status of itself as a profession. It has realised that the people it had to satisfy were local authorities who paid the bills, relatives who were relieved that somebody else was taking charge of their awkward members, and a public which did not understand mental troubles and was overawed by a display of scientific credentials. The fact that the psychiatric patients were too distressed, vulnerable, and ignorant to make a fuss added to the advantageous position of the profession. This is not the usual way of looking at a profession such as psychiatry. But when people complain about the actions of trades unions, they may overlook the fact that the psychiatric profession is one of the most successful trades unions in existence. It has not deserved to advance to the position it has attained, but it has been very skillful in getting there.

The psychiatric profession certainly engages in a lot of activity, and the public admires this. But the public particularly admires official activity. Voluntary activity does not command the same degree of admiration. If you do something for a friend, or bring him or her comfort, or save their life, you may gain praise, but you will not get prestige. Help given from friendship or kinship may in fact do more good to a person than anything they receive from official sources. But such activity does not have the standing of officially doing something for someone as part of a job.

There are many things about psychiatry which a large proportion of the public admires. There is hierarchy in psychiatric establishments. The psychiatrists are at the top. The clinical psychologists and the psychiatric social workers are below them. And the patients are at the bottom. The psychiatrists have a long period of training, since they have the same training as other doctors, but specialise in psychiatry in the last part of it. They do not have any compulsory training in psychotherapy. Any training in psychotherapy they have acquired has been entirely voluntary. This is in keeping with the adherence of official psychiatry to the medical model. Psychiatric establishments are run in a formal way. There is a lot of bureaucracy. Indeed, they are very similar to many other organisations in the outside world.

To most psychiatrists, the above is the correct way to do things, and many of the public would agree. The fact that this manner of proceeding is not appropriate for dealing with people in mental distress has not occurred to them, and it has not occurred to much of the public, either. It is interesting that many people who have experienced periods of mental distress get better without having recourse to official psychiatry at all. For some people, time itself does the work of healing. And this applies even to some of those who have experienced extreme mental distress. It is interesting, too, that many past psychiatric patients are very dissatisfied with the treatment they have received, and call themselves survivors.

Any requirement for biopsychiatrists to relate to their patients, to talk to them, and to take what they say seriously would represent a revolution in their whole mindset and in their whole professional life. It would mean that they would have to adopt new skills, which some may find difficult, and even fail. In some ways, their situation is similar to that of the handloom weavers at the start of the industrial revolution, though I have much more sympathy for the latter than for the biopsychiatrists.

If you think twice about it, it is absolutely absurd that somebody who specialises in dealing with mental patients with the professed aim of helping them should think it totally unnecessary to talk to them or ask them about their problems, and yet this is the reality with a great proportion of psychiatrists in practise today.

Freedom Of Choice

The freedom to practise the religion of your choice is enshrined in the laws of this country and of many other countries. If you say that particular beliefs, choices, and practices are part of your religion, then your right to act in accordance with them is granted. A Christian Scientist has every right to refuse medical treatment. A Jehovah's Witness can refuse to have blood transfusions. A Sikh motorcyclist is allowed to wear his turban rather than a crash helmet.

It could be argued strongly that wanting a particular type of mental health treatment, rather than another, if you have mental troubles, is really part of your religion. It is part of your religion, since it is part of your philosophy of life, and, quite frankly, it is very difficult to distinguish the two. Of course, if you are the only adherent of this philosophy of life, then it would be difficult to call it a religion, since a religion almost always involves a group of people. But this particular philosophy of life of yours could appeal to quite a number of people. Therefore, when you have collected a sizeable number of adherents, you could argue very strongly that you were an adherent of a religion, with all the rights and privileges pertaining to such.

If you have a bodily complaint or illness, you have complete rights to have the medical treatment of your choice or, alternatively, you can decide to have no treatment. The only restriction on your freedom is that some treatments might not be available on the NHS, meaning that you would have to pay for them. Another restriction is, if you are in an accident and are taken to the Accident And Emergency department of a hospital. It is generally assumed that you would want to be taken to such a place and treated after an accident. Now psychiatrists claim that their speciality is part of ordinary medicine. Therefore, logically, you should have the same freedom of choice as you would in ordinary medicine.

People who have been sectioned and subjected to unwelcome psychiatric treatment against their will could claim that their human rights have been infringed. Or if the people themselves are in no fit state to do this, their friends could claim this on their behalf. The existing law may not be in their favour, but the logic of their case is compelling. After all, human rights is supposed to be something which we are all keen on.

There are therfore, three grounds on which unwelcome psychiatric treatments could be called into question that they:-
1) Went against the principles of the person's religion.
2) Infringed on the person's right to a choice of medical treatment.
3) Were infringements of the person's human rights.

I do not know whether anybody thinks it worthwhile to pursue these further. But it is a thought!

Financial And Institutional Considerations

The profession of psychiatry has grown over the years to become part of the fabric of society.

If the notion of mental illness having a somatic cause is false, and if in fact there is no place for medicine in the field of mental troubles, then the appropriate people to deal with those with mental troubles, including psychotics, are psychotherapists, who need have no medical qualification at all. With regard to the referral of ordinary people by their general practitioners to a psychiatrist, they would now be referred to a psychotherapist instead. Those with genuine brain diseases or brain damage would be referred to neurologists. Violent criminals would be dealt with by the criminal law.

This could mean the end of the separate profession of psychiatry, since it appears to be bound up with the notion that mental troubles have an organic cause, and that they need physical or medical treatments to set them right.

The possibility would arise of a lot of people, unless they were also psychotherapists, either receiving money for retraining in something else, or receiving redundancy payments for early retirement. That is just the financial side of it. There is also the loss of prestige involved, which would be particularly disliked. However, possibly, since they must have acquired a certain amount of experience of different kinds of people in the course of their working lives, they could be employed in a consultative capacity, if they so wished. It would have to be on the clear understanding that their compulsory powers over people were a thing of the past.

With regard to the people employed as ancillary to the psychiatrists, such as psychiatric nurses, social workers, and clinical psychologists, they could most probably continue to be employed doing things not much different from what they are accustomed to.

The end of the profession of psychiatry would also mean that all those learned papers bolstering up the image of biopsychiatry would now be regarded as of very little value. And in so far as the medical profession itself has given support to the profession of psychiatry, it would have to endure the recognition that it had made a great mistake. Indeed, the whole scientific world would have to recognise that biopsychiatry was one of the biggest falsehoods in the history of science.

There is also the pharmaceutical industry to be considered. These companies were the manufacturers of the psychiatric drugs. This part of their business would very largely come to an end, or be seriously diminished. However, there is more than enough scope in the fields of ordinary medicine to make up for any losses incurred through giving up the manufacture and marketing of the psychiatric drugs. The loss in profits would be definitely short-term.

The end of institutional psychiatry as we know it would also have its impact on the attitudes of the general public. The latter would gradually have to think of what is called mental illness in a new way, realising that it is part of life, and could affect us all.

It is commonly thought that psychotherapy for all who wanted it, combined with a system of the prevalence of practical help and safe havens for all who needed them, would not be a viable proposition financially. I disagree. We do not live in a society where all public money is put to good use. The entire profession of psychiatry is ultimately dependant on the provision of public money. The money saved by the cessation of the need to train psychiatrists and pay them would be substantial. We must also remember that psychiatrists have to complete the entire medical training before they specialise in psychiatry. The training of psychoanalysts and psychothera-pists would not be as long, and so would cost less. Further, since the safe havens would not be run by mental health professionals but by ordinary people interested in helping the mentally distressed, and since they would be financed by voluntary contributions, there would also be financial savings in that area. The financial cost of psychiatric drugs is far from negligible. The accommodation of psychiatric patients in hospitals, together with the cost of their keep, is another item of public expenditure. In short, if you add up the total cost of the present state of affairs in mental health, you find that its abolition would be sufficient to finance the total cost of the proposals which I am advocating, including the cost of paying compensation to redundant psychiatrists. This way of thinking sounds idealistic. But there is another point. A person who is having psychotherapy is no more prevented from working than a person who is receiving medication, especially after the initial stages of severe incapacitating distress. Therefore, such a person is able to contribute to the cost of their treatment.

Further, existing public expenditure is not always devoted to necessary items. A great deal of the expenditure is made for idealistic reasons, which, on examination, do not produce any desirable results. We need to ask what the priorities of the public are, and to persuade more and more people of the justice of our cause.

There would probably have to be a gradual switch-over from the old way to the new way of doing things. And in the new way of doing things, the state should not directly finance anything to do with treatment, but should just ensure that people have enough money to pay for treatment if they so wish. In all this, the rôle of charitable donations and help would be very necessary.

Practical Proposals

We must realise that the intrusion of the medical model favoured by institutional psychiatry into the field of mental troubles is totally disastrous. People who have genuinely physical things wrong with their brains, either through injury or through disease, should see a neurologist. But for people who suffer from mental troubles, medicine has no legitimate rôle to play. It is overwhelmingly obvious that mental troubles are caused by the present or past environments to which a person has been subject, and the reactions of the person to these. Two things can be of help to a person with mental troubles. One is the improvement of their present life situation. And the other is psychotherapy, which aims to increase a person's awareness of past traumas, and to relive them, and thus to enable the person to evolve into a stronger personality as time passes.

Firstly, we must abolish the powers which psychiatrists have to section people, and force them to accept psychiatric treatments against their will.

Secondly, certain psychiatric treatments, such as lobotomy and ECT, should be outlawed entirely. It should be made a criminal offence to administer either of these treatments.

Thirdly, psychiatrists should also lose their powers with respect to the criminal law. The verdict of guilty but insane should be abolished. They should no longer be required to determine whether an accused was sane or not. The new system would leave any desirable leniency in a sentence to the discretion of the judge.

With regard to treatment, it must be understood that, for any treatment to have a chance of success, it must be entered into by the person receiving it entirely voluntarily. A person must want to be helped before he or she can be helped. Further, the treatment for mental troubles must be some kind of psychotherapy, or a mixture of therapies. It would be possible for someone to receive in-depth psychotherapy from one person, and some form of occupational therapy of their choice from another. But such treatment is in no way a quick fix for the person's problems. In the field of mental problems, as in life in general, there are no quick fixes.

In a previous chapter, the need for safe havens was recognised, where people with mental troubles could go if they wanted a period away from their usual surroundings. Those in a psychotic state could be encouraged to go there, but there should be no compulsion.

There is the question of whether drugs can form any part of a person's treatment for his or her problems. It is absolutely mandatory that drugs should not form a major part of the treatment. Any taking of drugs must be simply for the purpose of tidying someone over a period of very great distress. The dangers of the particular drug would need to be absolutely understood, and the length of time the person was on it would need to be short, and the dosage given the minimum possible. Any idea that a particular drug can target a particular mental disorder, and make it go away, should be utterly discarded. There might be a need for an advice centre which could give unbiased information as to what particular drugs actually do, and which drugs should be avoided absolutely.

The type of service, which consists of visiting the family of the person who is having the mental troubles, and trying to improve the family situation, has been done in a number of places, and has been a great help to both the individual and the family. This kind of work would continue as at present, and there could be more of it.

There is the question what should be done with the university departments of psychiatry, or the part of a general medical course devoted to psychiatry. Psychiatry would no longer be studied as a medical speciality. With regard to the university departments of psychiatry, there would have to be an investigation of what is taught, and of the academic literature produced, to see what was still relevant and useful, and what was not.

At present, institutional psychiatry is officially part of medicine. General practitioners regularly refer patients to psychiatrists if they think that their problems are psychological. Thus the medical profession colludes in the practices of psychiatry. Psychiatry is given a status which it would not have without it being regarded as part of medicine. Since, as we have seen, institutional psychiatry is far from benign, and is in fact dangerous, this reflects badly on the medical profession as a whole. Quite frankly, the medical profession would be better off if psychiatry was not part of it, if in fact institutional psychiatry as we know it were abolished. They could then refer people whose problems were psychological to psychotherapists.

There have been numerous instances over the years of people being destroyed, their lives completely wrecked, their minds mutilated by biopsychiatry. Morally, the biopsychiatrists responsible deserve the death penalty. At the very least, there should be some public acknowledgment of the terrible wrongs which were committed. But in actual fact, neither of these things will happen. In instances in history when there have been great wrongs, which are then abolished, it is often not expedient to punish people. On the contrary, it would probably be expedient to compensate a great many psychiatrists for loss of earnings. This is what happened when the act abolishing slavery in the British Empire was passed. The slave-owners were heavily compensated.

The implications of this book are that, effectively, institutional psychiatry should be abolished, since so much of what is damaging has been done in its name. However, having some knowledge of the way things are done in this country, a complete abolition may not happen. It will not matter too much, as long as the old ferocious teeth of psychiatry no longer bite.

18

Conclusion

The idea that there is a fundamentally wrong state of affairs in part of the life of the nation, and that this is supported by, or at least connived at, by the authorities will strike many people as almost incredible. The conventional wisdom is that we have got the basics right, and that wrongs of various sorts creep in when we translate our basics into practical activity.

But it is the contention of this book that we have got the basics wrong in the sphere of mental health by letting the whole thing be handled, as far as the state is concerned, by institutional psychiatry.

How could we have allowed this state of affairs to arise and continue?

There is the fact that many of us pay little attention to the minds of either ourselves or others. There is the deference to scientific authority. We allow institutional psychiatry, which has the support of the medical profession, to do our thinking for us, rather than investigate things for ourselves. There is the willingness to let certain of our fellow human beings be classified as fundamentally distinct from us, as happens with those classified as mentally ill.

We think that the persecution of witches happened in the past, and that nothing similar could happen in our country today. In fact, the damage done to people by biopsychiatry is very similar to the persecution of witches in the past. Both of them had a powerful ideology behind them. In the one case, the ideology was that witches existed, and could harm people by magical means. In the case of biopsychiatry, the ideology is that mental troubles are diseases which can be eradicated by physical or medical means. Both of these ideologies are false. There are similarities between the two cases. Witches were thought of as people apart from the rest of us, and so are people designated as mad. People were afraid of witches in the past, and, in some ways, they are afraid of the mentally disturbed today.

The view of mental illness as akin to bodily illness and caused in the same way is not only the viewpoint of the psychiatric establishment, but has also come to be the opinion of many of the general public. So not only does a war have to be waged against the former, but also the public outlook on mental illness has to change too.

The orthodox view has its attractions.

Firstly, it absolves everybody of any blame for mental illness. The nearest relatives are absolved for any behaviour of theirs which was harmful to their relative.

Secondly, the mentally ill person does not have to face painful memories from the past, and does not have to embark on the laborious journey to make sense of things, and work towards a better future. He or she can perhaps sink into a dependency condition, which may be congenial.

The abolition of institutional psychiatry as we know it is something which would principally affect those who might fall into its clutches. But it affects us all. As Abraham Lincoln implied in another context, you cannot have one dispensation for one set of people, and another dispensation for another set of people in the same country. Let us then look upon those in the clutches of institutional psychiatry as our brothers and sisters, and work with them, shoulder-to-shoulder, for the ending of the system.

We need to ask ourselves whether we really believe in the

liberties and values we claim to believe in. Do we really believe that human beings are fundamentally of equal importance? Do we really value the life of the mind, free from the effects of brain damage? Do we really value the full richness of human potential, unstunted, before it has a chance to reach fruition? Let us see the situation as it actually is, and strive with the utmost determination to change it. Let us cast aside the hesitations of biased experts and vested interests. Let us take up the cudgels for the sake of everyone, in order that they may enjoy the full human potential that some of us take for granted.

Ronald Bassman, "*A Fight To Be*" (2007)

Fred A. Baughman, "*The ADHD Fraud*" (2006)

Richard P. Bentall, "*Madness Explained, Psychosis And Human Nature*" (2003) and "*Doctoring The Mind*" (2009)

Susan Blackmore, "*The Meme Machine*" (1999)

Anton T. Boisen, "*The Exploration Of The Inner World*" (1936)

Mary Boyle, "*Schizophrenia, A Scientific Delusion?*" (1990)

Peter Breggin, "*Toxic Psychiatry*" (1993)

Paula J. Caplan, "*They Say You're Crazy*" (1995)

Axel Elof Carlson, "*The Unfit, A History Of A Bad Idea*" (2001)

Peter Chadwick, "*Understanding Parania*" (1995)

Leonard Roy Frank, "*The History Of Shock Treatment*" (1978)

George Frankl, "*The Failure Of The Sexual Revolution*" (1974), "*The Unknown Self*" (1990) and "*Exploring The Unconscious*" (1994)

Lester Grinspoon & James B. Bakalar, "*Psychedelic Drugs Reconsidered*" (1979)

Lucy Johnstone, "*Users And Abusers Of Psychiatry*" (1989)

Bertram P. Karon & Gary R. Vendenboss, "*Psychotherapy Of Schizophrenia*" (1981)

Helen Keller, "*The Story Of My Life*" (1947)

Herb Kutchins & Stuart R. Kirk, "*Making Us Crazy*" (1999)

Jeffrey Masson, "*Against Therapy*" (1989) and "*Final Analysis*" (1991)

Joanna Moncrief, "*The Myth Of This Chemical Cure*" (2008) and "*Psychiatric Drugs*" (2009)

Craig Newnes, Guy Holmes & Cailzie Dunn, "*This Is Madness*" (1999)

Richard B. Rosenbaum, "*Understanding Parkinson's Disease*" (2006)

Dorothy Rowe, "*Depression*" (1983) and "*Beyond Fear*" (1987)

Bertrand Russell, "*Power*" (1938)

Gilbert Ryle, "*The Concept Of Mind*" (1949)

Oliver Sacks, *"Awakenings"* (1973), *"The Man Who Mistook His Wife For A Hat"* (1985), *"An Anthropologist On Mars"* (1995) and *"Musicophilia"* (2008)
Susan Schaller, *"A Man Without Words"* (1991)
Andrew T. Scull, *"Museums Of Madness"* (1979)
David Shenk, *"The Forgetting"* (2001)
B.F. Skinner, *"Beyond Freedom And Dignity"* (1971)
Thomas Szasz, *"The Manufacture Of Madness"* (1971), *"The Myth Of Mental Illness"* (1972), *"Insanity The Idea And Its Consequences"* (1987) and *"Coercion As Cure"* (2007)
Thomas G. West, *"In The Mind's Eye"* (2009)

INDEX